Trauma-informed Care for Nurses and Allied Healthcare Professionals

This practical book equips nurses and healthcare practitioners with essential knowledge and skills for understanding and supporting people who are experiencing mental and emotional distress as a result of the unresolved effects of past trauma.

The book explores why people experiencing stress or distress due to adverse events in the distant or recent past, may use what are sometimes called 'maladaptive' coping mechanisms to relieve the intensity of their feelings. The skills-based approach of the book addresses key topics around adverse childhood events and trauma in ways that demonstrate the humanity of people living with mental health diagnoses or mental and emotional distress. Supporting readers to respond effectively and compassionately to people experiencing this type of distress, this book is informed throughout by anonymised service user perspectives and includes examples of good practice, suggestions for small changes that make meaningful differences and reflective activities.

Promoting practice that enables people who have experienced trauma to feel safer, more hopeful and function at their best, this guide is an essential read for all health professionals.

Sarah Housden is an occupational therapist and Associate Professor in Health Sciences at the University of East Anglia (UEA), passionate about improving healthcare practice for all.

Essential Mental Health Skills for Nurses and Allied Health Professionals
Series Editor: Sarah Housden

Trauma-Informed Care for Nurses and Allied Healthcare Professionals
Edited by Sarah Housden

Trauma-informed Care for Nurses and Allied Healthcare Professionals

Edited by
Sarah Housden

Routledge
Taylor & Francis Group

LONDON AND NEW YORK

Designed cover image: Getty Images

First published 2026
by Routledge
4 Park Square, Milton Park, Abingdon, Oxon OX14 4RN

and by Routledge
605 Third Avenue, New York, NY 10158

Routledge is an imprint of the Taylor & Francis Group, an informa business

For Product Safety Concerns and Information please contact our EU representative GPSR@taylorandfrancis.com. Taylor & Francis Verlag GmbH, Kaufingerstraße 24, 80331 München, Germany.

Trademark notice: Product or corporate names may be trademarks or registered trademarks, and are used only for identification and explanation without intent to infringe.

British Library Cataloguing-in-Publication Data
A catalogue record for this book is available from the British Library

ISBN: 978-1-041-06479-4 (hbk)
ISBN: 978-1-041-06478-7 (pbk)
ISBN: 978-1-003-63560-4 (ebk)

DOI: 10.4324/9781003635604

Typeset in Optima
by KnowledgeWorks Global Ltd.

Contents

List of figures   vii
List of tables   viii
Editor and contributor biographies   ix
Preface *by Sarah Housden*   x

1 **Introduction**   1
   Sarah Housden

2 **What is trauma?**   4
   Claire Moran

3 **The impact of adverse childhood experiences across
   the lifespan**   26
   Rebecca Turner

4 **Understanding and working with people with post-traumatic
   stress disorder**   41
   Hannah Bailey

5 **Effective support for people with complex PTSD and those
   diagnosed with a personality disorder**   61
   Sharon Martin-Brown

6 **Supporting traumatised individuals: Covering the B.A.C.E.S**   78
   Tamsin Black and Sarah Housden

7 **Health and care services and the risk of retraumatisation**   100
   Trudii Isherwood and Lou Cherrill

Contents

 8 **Trauma-informed care: Principles, practices and benefits**   **118**
    Hannah Bailey

 9 **The traumatised practitioner: Self-awareness, supervision
    and reflective practice**   **136**
    Sarah Housden

10 **Conclusion**   **155**
    Sarah Housden

Index   159

List of figures

4.1 Brain areas and structures influencing symptoms of PTSD   46
4.2 Picturing a tall window to support longer outbreaths   54

List of tables

4.1 Three groups of PTSD symptoms identified within ICD-11   48
8.1 An example of how TIC can change our response to
         perceived aggression   124
8.2 Three areas to build and develop in a TIC organisation   128

Editor and contributor biographies

Sarah Housden is Associate Professor in Health Sciences at the University of East Anglia and an occupational therapist by background.

Hannah Bailey is a mental health nurse with expertise in delivering therapeutic interventions for people who have lived experience of trauma.

Tamsin Black is Consultant Clinical Psychologist and ELFT Psychological Therapies Lead at the East London NHS Foundation Trust.

Lou Cherrill is an academic and researcher and continues to work in community mental health as a specialist mental health nurse with experience in delivering dialectical behavioural therapy.

Trudii Isherwood is a mental health nurse with a Master's degree in Advanced Practice and is accomplished delivering change in practice to reduce patient and service user retraumatisation.

Sharon Martin-Brown is an experienced mental health nurse working largely in the field of supporting people with emotional dysregulation.

Claire Moran is a lecturer in occupational therapy at UEA, with expertise in psychotherapeutic interventions for people who have experienced trauma across the lifespan.

Rebecca Turner is a nurse, clinical educator and doctoral student who is undertaking research into nurses' understanding of adverse childhood events.

Preface

'*Essential Mental Health Skills for Nurses and Allied Health Professionals*' offers a series of books on key topics aimed at equipping non-specialist mental health practitioners with knowledge, skills and understanding about the causes of mental and emotional distress, alongside tools for responding to people in their care who may be distressed or at risk of coming to harm due to a deterioration in their mental health.

Mental health presentations are increasingly evident across all areas of health and care provision, while specialist mental health services sometimes find it difficult to manage and respond to growing expressions of need amongst the population. This has resulted in an exponential growth in the demands made on general health and care practitioners to respond to people in mental and emotional distress, often in the absence of the timely availability of specialist mental health services with capacity to respond swiftly.

Within this series, readers will be able to explore the interplay between a variety of factors contributing to mental ill-health as they reflect on case studies of people with lived experience. These case studies are provided alongside more theoretical content and practical tools for immediate use, as well as information on more specialist therapeutic approaches and longer-term strategies for improving services. Theoretical ideas with examples of application to practice, followed by questions for reflection and discussion, provide practitioners, students and educators with opportunities to consider their own values and beliefs in the light of research, theory and evidence-based practice.

While acknowledging the challenges of contemporary healthcare practice, the series aims to support health and care practitioners to better understand the viewpoints of service users, and thus to move towards developing a more empathic and compassionate approach to working with people living with mental health-related illnesses and other signs of stress and distress.

The books in this series are written for nurses and allied health professionals who are seeking an enhanced understanding of mental health to support their ongoing professional development as well as their clinical practice with patients and service users who are experiencing distress. It has been one of the highlights of my career as an academic, which I hope to enhance through this book series, to see health practitioners of all professions come to new understandings of people experiencing mental distress, leading to more empathic and compassionate approaches to healthcare delivery.

It is equally important to note that the world of healthcare is not neatly divided into people who have mental health problems and those who are here to support them. There is no 'us' and 'them' in healthcare: health practitioners are just as likely to have experienced trauma and to be living with mental distress, as those with whom they work. This is reflected in the fact that many of us who have authored chapters within this series are people who have a mixture of expertise by experience (as carers and service users) alongside being people who have acquired expertise through study and by working as healthcare practitioners, researchers and academics. It is also worth noting that some of the case studies in this series are written by the editing and authorship team, based on our anonymised personal experiences as service users. This moves us beyond a tokenistic inclusion of the voices of service users to the meaningful production of a series of books that integrate service user expertise, just as it is integrated into our everyday lives and workplaces.

Dr Sarah Housden
Series Editor
June 2025

Introduction

Sarah Housden

As the first book in the *'Essential Mental Health Skills for Nurses and Allied Health Professionals'* series, the focus on trauma and trauma-informed care (TIC) within this book addresses an area of practice where nurses and allied health professionals can often find themselves feeling uncertain about the root causes of patient and service user actions. This includes how best to respond to patients expressing and experiencing high levels of emotional distress.

There is a growing need for mental health services to address the needs of people experiencing mental and emotional distress, which often arises from the unresolved effects of adverse childhood events (ACEs) or more recent traumatic events, for which symptoms can take the form of intense 'flash-backs' to past experiences. Other signs of post-traumatic stress include high levels of anxiety and corresponding vigilance with alertness to danger in the present even where there may be no current risk. However, a growth in the need for support for traumatised individuals, has not been matched by a corresponding growth in the resourcing of specialist services.

This book aims to enable healthcare practitioners of all professions to increase their knowledge and understanding of people experiencing stress or distress due to adverse events in the distant or recent past. The book aims to equip nurses and allied health professionals across settings to be effective, understanding and compassionate in their responses to people living with mental or emotional distress, who may be in their care for reasons other than their mental health.

This book addresses key issues around ACEs and trauma in ways that demonstrate the humanity of people living with mental health diagnoses or mental and emotional distress. There can be considerable anxiety amongst

DOI: 10.4324/9781003635604-1

non-specialist health and care professionals about working with people who are traumatised and whose mental health diagnoses may lead to them being stigmatised within general health and care provision. This book aims to equip healthcare practitioners to respond effectively to expressions of trauma and distress, and therefore begins to address some of the key areas of need facing health and care services today. Our aim is that, when the ideas here are implemented, people with trauma of diverse origins can feel safer, experience hope and function at their best both whilst receiving services and in other settings.

As you read, you will notice that the terminology used to describe those who live with mental and emotional distress, includes terms such as service user, patient and survivor. Although for practical purposes, a decision needed to be made to adopt some form of specific descriptive term, we would not want anyone to feel defined by these descriptions and believe that all people have the right to describe their relationship to service providers and to their own experiences, in whatever way feels most comfortable and appropriate to them. As authors, we also believe that there is no 'them' and 'us' in healthcare as we all have the potential to become patients and service users at some point in our lives.

Claire Moran begins the book with an exploration of what trauma is in Chapter 2, closely followed by further examination of ACEs with Rebecca Turner in Chapter 3. In the next two chapters, Hannah Bailey enhances readers' understanding of post-traumatic stress disorder (PTSD), including the physiological processes involved in a single trauma event, and Sharon Martin-Brown focuses on complex post-traumatic stress disorder (C-PTSD), which can occur where trauma has been multiple-event or sustained. Tamsin Black's focus in Chapter 6 moves to how a person can be supported to recover from and manage the effects of trauma, both through therapy and by strengthening some fundamental approaches to regaining and maintaining wellbeing. Chapter 7, by Trudii Isherwood and Lou Cherrill, explores the risks of retraumatisation and ways of minimalising such risks. This is complemented by Hannah Bailey's review of TIC and consideration of the different elements of TIC and its implementation in everyday nursing and healthcare practice. The final main chapter consists of a consideration of the needs of practitioners as people who may have experienced traumas themselves at some point, but also as people who are at risk of exposure to moral, vicarious and secondary traumas in their everyday work. The book then rounds off with key points for best practice that are aimed at being straightforward enough for most nurses and healthcare practitioners to implement, regardless of workplace and organisational context.

Within each of these chapters, there is a case study based on real events and experiences of someone known either to the author or to another member of the authorship and editorial team. Aimed at being illustrative as well as supporting the application of theory to practice, these case studies enhance understanding of real-world issues and bring the text into the reality of everyday practice.

Another key focus within Chapters 2–8 is the inclusion of a 'Tools for Now' section, which provides ideas for small changes in our practice and approach, which can make a big difference to service users. These sections are followed with considerations around longer-term treatments and interventions for which individuals could be referred, as well as ideas for organisations and managers focused on the strategic implementation of trauma-informed approaches to practice.

It is hoped that this book, along with other volumes in the '*Essential Mental Health Skills for Nurses and Allied Health Professionals*' series, will play a key role in the education and professional development of nurses and allied health professionals going forward. The development of knowledge, understanding and skills for practice will be enhanced through readers' active engagement with the questions for reflection and discussion, together with the suggestions for further reading, towards the end of each chapter. These will, ideally, be used for personal as well as team reflection and follow-up learning.

The authors and editor have produced this book in the hope that it will make a difference to you in promoting confidence and advancing your competence in interacting with people who have experienced trauma. Ultimately, our aim is that this will in turn lead to benefits for you, your service users and patients, for the teams you are part of and for the organisations for which you work.

What is trauma?

Claire Moran

Case study

Ashley's story

Looking back, it is difficult to pinpoint a precise occasion when I first experienced what I would now call abuse at the hands of another person. I guess in some ways, it started with emotional neglect, which meant that I never really learnt to respect and value myself or to put appropriate boundaries in place. The boundaries, now, look like a big part of it. I wanted so much to be loved by my family, and to have a sense of belonging, that when my older brother, Jack, invited me to jump into bed with him to keep warm, I hardly thought twice about whether I wanted to do it. He wanted me to snuggle up with him, and that was the closest I'd come in a very long time, to anyone wanting to be with me or spend time with me.

Actually, it was probably the closest thing to receiving a show of affection I'd ever had. It was okay that first time. He touched bits of me that I knew were meant to be kept private, but he didn't hurt me. I really did feel loved and wanted. Things changed gradually, over the coming weeks, becoming more intimate. Then one day, Dad walked in on us and there was one almighty row. My brother moved out that evening to sofa-surf with friends, and we gradually lost touch with him altogether. I was left feeling emotionally bewildered, with neither Mum or Dad being willing to talk to me

DOI: 10.4324/9781003635604-2

about Jack, and me not daring to mention anything about what had happened with him to friends at school. I felt abhorrent to my family and didn't want anyone else knowing about what I had done, for fear of losing their friendships.

By the time I reached late teens, I was getting what I'd call properly interested in boys and had a few boyfriends in fairly quick succession. I was pretty much happy for them to treat me as they liked, without objecting to parts of my body being handled by relative strangers, after them not seeing the light of day since my experiences with Jack. It was easy enough getting on the contraceptive pill and for a time I settled for a life of short relationships with little emotional engagement. I hardly got chance to say much more than 'hello' before most of the men I was acquainted with would lead me to the bedroom. Somewhere deep inside I knew that I was worth more than this, but it did seem in line with what I knew of the relationships some of my friends were having at the time, so I put these sexual encounters down to something I would have to learn to put up with. It seemed to me to be part of what it meant to be a woman. Even so, I felt like I was being handled like a bag of potatoes, or as I secretly thought of myself, a lump of meat whose feelings were unrecognised.

I was in my early twenties when I first said 'no' to one of the men who wanted to have sex with me. This led very quickly, within moments it seemed, to a beating and being raped. Only I didn't see it as rape, as much as the natural conclusion to a miserable life story. I certainly never reported what had happened as rape and could hear my internalised judge, if the case was brought to court, saying: 'what did you expect?'.

I stopped going out after that, and steered clear of friends who enjoyed pubbing and clubbing as I felt like there was something about me which attracted abuse. Instead, I spent the evenings watching telly and only went out when work required me to – a necessity to pay the rent on my flat. I felt so worthless and was fearful of ever having a relationship with a man again.

I can't exactly say what led to the decision to end my life a few months later. What I can say is that my somewhat rough handling by some staff at the local emergency department, alongside the quickly fired questions from their mental health liaison team, left me in no frame of mind to talk about my experiences. So, I was sent home to try taking my life again, and again, until five years later when someone gave me the time and space to begin to share and understand my life story, and to start the long process of healing through learning to love and care for myself.

Introduction

The word 'trauma' has become ubiquitous in the English language over the last decade or so, thanks in part perhaps to the prevalence of its colloquial use across social media platforms. Originating from the Greek meaning 'a wound, a hurt, a defeat', the contemporary use of the word trauma has been increasingly associated with psychological harm. The language and labels we choose have powerful effects, and the recognition of psychological trauma perhaps reflects a sociocultural shift, in which psychological 'wounds' are being recognised in our cultural lexicon.

Chapter aims

This chapter focusses on providing a detailed and comprehensive overview of trauma and includes information and ideas which seek to explore:

- What causes trauma and the aspects of trauma contributing to long-term psychological harm.
- Different types of trauma and the damaging effect of neglect.
- Wider societal patterns of inequality and disadvantage which can contribute to the lasting effects of traumatic experiences.
- Recognising our role in supporting people to share their story and to move towards recovery.

What is trauma?

Let's start by imagining that trauma is a normal reaction to a significant event – something which is emotionally distressing and causing pain. The *Diagnostic and Statistical Manual of Mental Disorders*, 5th Edition (DSM-5-TR) (APA, 2022) defines traumatic events as exposure to actual or threatened death, serious injury or sexual violence through direct experience, witnessing or learning about violent or accidental traumas that have occurred for close family members or friends. Childhood trauma may include physical, sexual or psychological neglect and abuse, disasters or terrorism, family or community violence, bereavement and serious accidents or life-threatening illness (National Child Traumatic Stress Network, 2020). The World Health Organization (WHO) estimated that in 2014, approximately 36%, 22% and 16% of children worldwide have experienced emotional abuse, physical abuse and neglect, respectively. Some researchers define two different types of trauma, namely: 'event trauma' which is a sudden, unexpected traumatic event such as an accident; and 'process trauma' which is a continued exposure to a long-lasting stressor, such as war or physical abuse (Shaw, 2000).

The contemporary western mental health system is characterised as being diagnostic led. There are several diagnoses associated with trauma, such as post-traumatic stress disorder (PTSD), complex PTSD, developmental trauma disorder (DTD), attachment disorder and emotionally unstable personality disorder (EUPD). All these diagnoses share a collection of symptoms including emotional dysregulation, somatic symptoms and interpersonal difficulties, alongside cognitive and behavioural difficulties. As nurses and allied health professionals (AHPs) practising in a holistic and person centred way, our interest should be in the individual and the symptoms we see in front of us, and their current presentation, focussing on how we might be able to help to alleviate those symptoms, regardless of diagnosis.

The Centre for Disease Control Adverse Childhood Experiences (ACEs) (Felitti et al., 1998) study was a seminal project, exploring the myriad impacts of psychological trauma across the lifespan by surveying historical health outcomes of 17,000 individuals in California. They found a direct link between childhood trauma and the onset of chronic disease, imprisonment and even unemployment in adults. The original questionnaire indicated ACEs in three areas: abuse (emotional, sexual, physical), neglect (physical, emotional) and household dysfunction (mental illness, imprisoned family member, witnessing violence towards mother, substance abuse, divorce). The study found that the presence of four or more ACEs was linked to early mortality. In the context of the United Kingdom, the Office for National Statistics (ONS, 2020) indicates that one in five adults aged 18–74 years (8.5 million people) experienced at least one form of child abuse before the age of 16, whether this was emotional, physical or sexual in nature, or involved witnessing domestic violence.

To qualify as adverse events, McLaughlin et al. (2019) noted that experiences of threat or deprivation must either be chronic or involve single events that are severe enough to require significant emotional, cognitive or neurobiological adaptation by an average child (for example, sexual abuse). There is extensive empirical literature on the relationship between the cumulative number of ACEs and mental health difficulties (Hogg et al., 2023). Furthermore, the idea of cumulative risk modelling acknowledges the impact of multiple adverse experiences on a person, impacting their ability to process future adverse events (Oral et al., 2016).

Researchers have found a relationship between adverse experiences and behavioural problems amongst children and adolescents, anxiety disorders, depression and suicide attempts. Four or more ACEs increased the risk of depression (4.5 times) and suicide attempts (12.2–15.3 times) (Felitti et al., 1998; Hogg et al., 2023). However, Kelly-Irving and Delpierre (2019) offer a critique on ACEs, acknowledging that although the literature surrounding ACEs was a helpful move towards recognition of psychological trauma, ACEs cannot be removed from the wider socioeconomic landscape. The original ACE study did not account for wider social experiences such as racism and sexism, instead focussing on trauma within the household. For context, subsequent research details that people from black and ethnic minority groups are likely to die younger due to social circumstances (ONS, 2020) and also receive poorer treatment in the healthcare system (Hamed et al., 2022). These are significant systemic traumas that were not included in the original ACEs questionnaire.

There is a need for a wider definition of ACEs as many research participants report stressful experiences that are not included on the original scale, but which are likely to belong in the same category (Finkelhor et al., 2015). Examples include social isolation and victimisation, as well as perceived discrimination. Further forms of adversity described in the literature include bereavement, sudden and frequent relocations, serious accidents, life-threatening childhood illness, pornography (exposure to or participation in), prostitution, natural disasters, kidnapping, torture, war, refugee camps and terrorism (Oral et al., 2016).

Adverse experiences are also related to poverty. The United Kingdom has one of the highest rates of child poverty in Europe (Bradshaw, 2023). A recent WHO and UN report detailed that mental health difficulties are mostly determined by social factors, rather than biochemistry (WHO and United Nations, 2023). Marmot et al. (2020) indicate that health inequalities have increased in the United Kingdom and that life expectancy has stalled. Climate change is another emerging global context that can result in frequent traumatic experiences due to disaster exposure and unplanned migration (Olff et al., 2025).

Defining trauma explicitly is complex as the subjective interpretation of an experience can be more relevant that the objective facts of the event, meaning that it is not necessarily the trauma itself, but the sense that we make of it, which can be psychologically and emotionally damaging in the long term. This involves recognising the role played by the emotions and thoughts associated with the event, along with the cumulative effect on a person, which itself can depend on a multitude of factors, both personal and systemic. In a narrative review of 15 years of psychotraumatology, Olff et al. (2025) noted that there is no universal experience or response to trauma. They found that symptoms experienced following trauma differ depending on the age and developmental phase, sex and gender, sociocultural and environmental contexts of the individual, as well as on systemic socio-political forces. Furthermore, the effects of trauma may be mitigated by, and depend on, levels of resilience and access to social support, as well as the educational attainment of individuals and the social groups to which they belong.

This becomes pertinent in practice for nurses and AHPs, because it signifies that we would do well not to assume the meaning or impact of trauma for an individual. Instead, we must remain open and curious to the person in front of us in every healthcare encounter.

Traumatic experiences

Attachment, relational and developmental trauma

Research has consistently demonstrated that complex interpersonal trauma has a severe impact on the developing child when it happens in the context of attachment (George, 2025; Lucre et al., 2024). Attachment is a clinical term used to describe the lasting psychological connectedness between human beings (Bowlby, 1969). To survive and thrive, attachment and connection with caregivers is essential. A growing brain needs a supportive environment and language acquisition, emotionally attentive caregivers, adequate nutrition and *some* stress, termed 'eustress' – stress which is believed to have positive effects on health and performance (Shonkoff et al., 2012).

Human beings are distinct from other animals in that infants remain immature and dependent on their mothers for much longer than other primates and are slower to attain developmental milestones such as walking (Rosenberg, 2021). The result is that infant brains grow rapidly while experiencing a richer sensory and social environment than they would have, if following the typical developmental course of a primate (Bjorklund, 2022). The malleable brain plasticity of an infant allows for dynamic responses to the socio-emotional environment they are born into, with repeated interactions and communications supporting memory-making and laying the foundation for relationships. Vygotsky's (1978) social learning theory understands human development as being a socially mediated process, by which children acquire cultural beliefs, values and strategies from their surrounding environment, including their caregivers. The early years of an infant's life are seen as a 'window of opportunity' as well as a 'point of vulnerability' (Andersen, 2003), while other research has demonstrated that the first two years of a child's life are the most critical for forming attachments (Prior and Glaser, 2006).

Humans are relational beings – we exist in relation to ourselves, to others and to the wider sociocultural environment of family, friends, workplaces, the government and the natural world in which we live. The complexity of the human experience means that while we are compelled towards connection and cooperation, we are also vulnerable to interpersonal harm. A child or adolescent is dependent upon their caregivers for safety and security, nurture and care. The process of healthy attachment involves micro-traumas whereby a child might hurt themselves and become distressed and the caregiver soothes the child. The attachment bond is thereby strengthened. Sometimes, the caregiver perhaps cannot attend to the child in time, but this is survivable in a consistent, loving environment – it is *good enough* (Winnicott, 2000).

However, in environments where caregivers are not present, or are a frightening presence, the child has no choice but to attach, for purposes of survival, to a caregiver who is causing them harm. Living in fear and relying on this caregiver for such things as food and shelter result in prolonged exposure to chronic stress, which impacts the brain and behaviour as well as subsequent attachments. The necessity of this dependence on an unreliable caregiver can result internally in mixing up concepts of care and love with those of abuse and neglect, the effects of which can last a lifetime.

Often, the adults we see in mental health services have been victims of childhood trauma. As opposed to PTSD, often associated with an event trauma, such as an experience of war (see Chapter 4), complex PTSD (C-PTSD) is a diagnosis associated with trauma in the context of relational attachment, in a trusted relationship (see Chapter 5 for further information).

The experience of relational or attachment trauma can have a deeply profound effect and impact on future relational experiences. Bowlby (1969) referred to this as the 'internal working model of the self' and proposed that the attachment styles learned in early childhood form a model for future attachments into adulthood. Childhood trauma may serve as a template for future relational patterns with caregiver-like figures encountered during adulthood (Selwyn et al., 2021). This can manifest in repeated abusive relationships, as a compulsion towards a known model of relationships that feels familiar. An example of this is seen in the case study of Ashley, who experiences repeated abusive and emotionally neglectful relationships through adolescence, following a relatively early childhood trauma of sexual abuse which becomes associated with self-blame and a poor sense of bodily autonomy. It is not only the amount of trauma, but also the nature of the trauma exposure that has a relationship with one's self-concept. This is supported by findings in the research literature concerning adults, which suggests that child sexual abuse is linked to worse outcomes later in life, relative to other trauma exposure types (Maniglio, 2009).

Trauma begets trauma, meaning the experiencing of relational traumatic events are implicated in further traumatic events across the lifespan. Notably, the nature and intensity of the effects of trauma on a person greatly depend on the type and timing of these events during sensitive developmental periods (Tomoda et al., 2024). Adolescence, between 10 and 19 years, is a sensitive period for brain development. It is therefore helpful to know when trauma took place. Childhood maltreatment that occurs earlier in life and continues for a longer duration is associated with the worst outcomes (Dunn et al., 2018).

Emotional abuse is pervasive and can include many things, such as controlling behaviours, manipulation, invalidation and constant criticism.

Hoeboer et al. (2021) found that emotional abuse, as opposed to any other form of maltreatment, was associated with more severe PTSD symptoms. The association between exposure to childhood trauma and mental health outcomes is found to be larger in those with greater exposure, with a particularly increased risk for those exposed to emotional abuse and neglect (Humphreys et al., 2020). Childhood emotional abuse is implicated in insecure attachment styles, alongside difficulties in identity formation, intimacy and empathy, as well as symptoms of hopelessness, substance abuse, psychosis and borderline personality disorder (Spinazzola et al., 2021). Emotional abuse can be challenging to identify and evidence, due to its insidious nature and the invisibility of the wounds.

The trauma of neglect

Whereas emotional, physical and sexual abuse could be conceived of as being done to a person, neglect can perhaps be characterised as a chronic absence of doing the things which are needed for healthy development. It is empty space where love should be. Neglect in the very early stage of development can have catastrophic effects on attachment and child development. To survive and thrive, a child needs connection, nourishment and language. Without these, brain and social development is impacted (Lyons-Ruth et al., 2023).

Neglect can take on various forms in modern society, including physical neglect, such as not having enough food to eat and warm clothes, or neglect of the home environment, including lack of hygiene or hoarding. Emotional neglect can involve not feeling listened to, heard or believed by caregivers.

It is now known that neglect is associated with neurocognitive alterations, impairing psychosocial functioning and increased risk of developing psychiatric disorders (2023). Carvalho Silva et al. (2024) emphasise the need for paying increased attention to the effects of neglect on children, due to its impact on health outcomes across the lifespan. Neglect has been found to be the strongest risk factor for developing major depressive disorder or depressive symptoms, particularly in females, in comparison to other types of maltreatment (Carvalho Silva et al., 2024). In England, the number of looked after children has increased every year since 2008, and most children in care are there due to abuse or neglect (NSPCC, 2024a). Looked after children are also more likely to have a mental health issue, and lower levels of wellbeing (Miller et al., 2023).

Neglect also features as a symptom of alcohol and substance misuse, impacting dependants. Estimated figures for children of alcoholics (COAs) in the United Kingdom are in excess of 70,000 (NSPCC, 2024b) and link to there being in excess of 600,000 dependent drinkers in England (Alcohol Change, 2018). The nature of alcohol and drug use leads to an unreliable caregiver who may oscillate from extreme high moods to absence and sleeping all day.

To extend our understanding of neglect, we might also consider the experience of individuals within a neglectful system. With 4.3 million children, or 30% of all children in the UK, living in poverty (House of Lords, UK Parliament, 2024). With cuts in state benefits in recent years, including for some of the most vulnerable in society, alongside issues associated with social determinants of health linked to class and racism, it is essential to consider the wider systemic trauma experienced by a person existing in a world that appears to discriminate against them consistently.

Systemic/structural trauma

Systemic trauma refers to experiences of oppression, discrimination and prejudice based on the systems surrounding us, which are associated with the politics of power. This could refer to disability, gender or ethnicity, for example, and is a vital consideration when working with patients and service users.

Structural racism can include not only interpersonal acts of discrimination, but also wider socioeconomic structures, maintained through prejudice, discrimination, policies, practices, social norms and the structures of wider society. Health inequalities more clearly impact ethnic minoritised individuals, such as higher mortality rates in the healthcare system, notably exacerbated by COVID-19 (Essex et al., 2022). Racial trauma is also likely to be under-reported due to lack of awareness or bias amongst clinicians and discomfort in discussing these issues (Kirkinis et al., 2018). In addition to this, children are more likely to be taken into care if they are male and of black or mixed ethnicity (NSPCC, 2024a).

In terms of gender discrimination, the National Policing Statement (2024), recorded over one million crimes related to Violence Against Women and Girls (VAWG) during 2022–2023, accounting for 20% of all police-recorded crime. There was also an increase of 37% in recorded VAWG-related crime between 2018 and 2023. Males are more likely to experience non-sexual assault and combat-related trauma, while females are more likely to be exposed to sexual assault and childhood sexual abuse (Dalvie and Daskalakis, 2021).

It is also helpful to consider the differences in gendered responses by diagnosing clinicians to people who have experienced traumatic events. In our current medically focussed diagnostic system, women are more likely to receive a diagnosis of emotionally unstable personality disorder or border-line personality disorder than men, with these diagnoses often being asso-ciated with experiences of childhood trauma. By contrast, men are more likely to receive a diagnosis of anti-social behaviour disorder and are more likely to be imprisoned – with prisoners often reporting high levels of child-hood trauma (Wolff and Shi, 2012).

Effects of trauma

Physiological responses

Research has demonstrated that trauma or stress experienced during child-hood and adulthood increases the risk of developing psychopathology such as post-traumatic stress disorder and depression (Dalvie and Daskalakis, 2021). Understandings of the body's stress response suggest that it is a complex and integrative process that involves, neuronal–neuroendocrine–immune interactions and that these interactions are also influenced by an individual's genetic background. Adverse patterns of social experiences – such as neglect and abuse – are associated with atypical structural and functional brain fea-tures (McLaughlin et al., 2019), while exposure to chronic stress can induce neuronal remodelling and is associated with increased anxiety and PTSD symptomology (McEwen, 2019).

Exposure to the threat of trauma stimulates the autonomic nervous system (ANS), resulting in hyperarousal states accompanying survival responses such as fight, flight, submission and freeze (see, for example, Siegel, 2006). Responses can include those which go beyond the traditionally identified 'fight or flight':

- Freeze – feeling paralysed or unable to move
- Flop – doing what you're told without being able to protest
- Fight – fighting, struggling or protesting
- Flight – hiding or moving away

- Fawn – trying to please someone who harms you
- Faint – succumbing to a horizontal position whereby blood supply increases to the brain

These bodily responses to threats and stressors have biologically evolved to enable survival. However, a household where the threat is unremitting and in the context of dependence on attachment figures, this will lead to chronic stress on bodily systems and presentations of mental distress with symptoms such as hypervigilance and heightened responses on exposure to triggers, even at times where the threat is not acute. The combination of the over-appraisal of the threat, alongside the self-assessment of inability to cope, results in potentially extreme emotional reactions to any perceived threat.

It is also important to note that for many trauma survivors, the body can become a source of pain, intrusion and shame. Survivors may therefore feel disconnected from their bodies and from their reactions to stressors.

Emotional dysregulation and mental health outcomes

Childhood is characterised by elevated neural plasticity and developing neurobiological systems, and therefore, chronic stress in childhood appears to effect emotions and the mediation of stress responses later in life, increasing the risk for psychological distress presenting as psychiatric disorders (Olff et al., 2025). Extensive research has demonstrated a link between childhood trauma and mood disorders (for example, Galatzer-Levy et al., 2018; Melamed et al., 2024; Winston and Chicot, 2016). One meta-analysis revealed that 46% of individuals with depression report childhood maltreatment (Nelson et al., 2017).

One of the notable effects of interpersonal trauma appears to be emotional instability, which may materialise in various ways, such as suicide attempts, self-harm, relationship difficulties and even physical health issues. Traumatic events may have a wide range of transdiagnostic mental and physical health consequences, not limited to post-traumatic stress disorder (Olff et al., 2025). Altered patterns of emotional, cognitive and social development have been observed consistently amongst children who have experienced adversity (McLaughlin et al., 2019).

Understanding the impact of trauma on the brain and relational behaviour calls into question the diagnostic approach taken by modern-day mental healthcare systems. A psychiatry-led system results in a reliance on the medical model of health – when so often what we are seeing is, realistically, a normal response to abnormal and damaging circumstances.

Nurses and AHPs working in emergency departments will experience attendance by those who have tried to take their lives more often than is the case for health practitioners working in other settings. Past trauma may show itself in patients with substance misuse issues, relationship difficulties, inability to stay in employment or interactions with service providers which come across as challenging.

It is also helpful to consider somatic symptomology. Given that many health practitioners work across physical and mental health settings, it is essential to be aware that we may come across patients with somatic symptoms. These are physical problems that do not have an identifiable physiological origin, causing significant stress and functional impairment to the individual (Greenman et al., 2024). Patients presenting with medically unexplained symptoms are prevalent in healthcare, accounting for around 45% of all GP consultations (Jadhakhan et al., 2022). Kratzer et al. (2022) linked symptoms of hyperarousal seen in patients with somatic symptoms, with a biopsychosocial understanding of childhood trauma, noting that early bodily experiences of chronic stress may lead to later over-appraisal of physical symptoms. It can be helpful to consider trauma as a transdiagnostic vulnerability factor when working with patients experiencing fatigue, pain and other physical issues. Research continues to explore this area.

However, it is both helpful and hopeful to note that the most common response to trauma is resilience. In a narrative review of research focussing on trauma, Olff et al. (2025) identified moderating factors that may be able to differentiate between trajectories of risk and resilience, and found that aspects of emotional functioning, such as coping flexibility, coping strategies and style, perceived self-efficacy, optimism, neuroticism and resilience beliefs, play potentially significant roles.

Why is understanding trauma important for health professionals?

Working in modern healthcare means that we will come across various forms of trauma – not only as a clinician treating our patients, but also, perhaps, as a victim ourselves. A health practitioner working in the emergency department might see repeated attendance of some people, due to suicidal ideation and actions. In these moments, there is a danger that the stigma in the system might result in not treating these patients with the care they need.

An important consideration in terms of the service user's emotional response to trauma is shame. Shame can be conceived as a global devaluation of the self (Budiarto and Helmi, 2021). Unfortunately, shame has sometimes been used in clinical practice, to reprimand people who have harmed themselves or experienced suicidal thoughts and actions. Given the likelihood of service users having an existing trauma-derived sense of shame, this approach from a health professional can be devastatingly detrimental to the long-term recovery of the individual. Hence, in the case study of Ashley, we see a five-year journey of repeated self-harming before someone takes a non-judgemental approach to understanding and listening.

Patients remember those who are kind to them, who listen and who do not make them feel ashamed. Some patients experience systemic healthcare trauma from services. This can take the form of not being believed or not being listened to, resulting in a complex relationship with healthcare providers which can lead to feelings of suspicion, and a reluctance to engage, combined with a fear of authority. (Chapter 8 provides further information on the risks associated with re-traumatisation.)

Most healthcare professionals experience increasing complexity in their caseloads within contemporary healthcare practice. Given the extent of traumatic experiences across the population, amidst the backdrop of systemic inequalities, it is likely we will frequently meet traumatised patients. However, equipped with the knowledge and understanding of cause and effect, we are better able to validate patients and support them to get the help they need.

Tools for now: small changes that can make a big difference

All health practitioners need to be aware of the need to sensitively signpost service users and patients to services which are likely to be of most help to them, doing this in a way which emphasises your understanding of what they have experienced.

1. Be aware that you and your colleagues may also have experienced trauma of some kind (see Chapter 9 for further information). Pay attention to your own history and experiences, seeking to learn ways in which

to protect yourself. Developing self-awareness and resilience through reflection along with discussions with a trusted colleague, friend or family member, are useful facets of this.

2. Listen to and remain curious about the stories of patients and service users, listening to their narratives with open and empathic responses. Working with people who have experienced trauma is not so much about identifying what is wrong with a person, as listening to their stories of survival and recovery.

3. It may be possible to introduce sensitive approaches to screening for trauma histories in settings such as the emergency department, through validated questionnaires, clinical interviews and discussion with the service user, or by reviewing past patient records. This can give us a better understanding of the wider issues that might bring people back to our services and in some cases, avoid the risks associated with re-traumatising people.

4. Listen to service users and patients, supporting them as they find words to express what has happened or is happening for them.

5. Offer validation to service users and patients, recognising that past experiences of health and care systems may have damaged them and that winning the trust of traumatised individuals takes time. Be especially aware that past experiences of shaming within healthcare settings, and fear of this being repeated, may be contributing to how the person is presenting in the moment.

6. Recognise that you can make a significant difference just by demonstrating compassion, kindness and empathy. You don't need to know all the details of an individual's story to be able to care. Listen to what they are willing to share without asking intrusive questions.

7. Be mindful that traumas which occurred in childhood and adolescence have an impact across the lifespan. A person's age does not exclude them from the ongoing effects of early life traumas, and it is worth noting that incidence of suicide amongst older adults (over 65s) is correlated with adverse childhood events (Sachs-Ericsson et al., 2016)

Reducing and managing trauma: systemic and longer-term approaches

Research helps explain how some people are able to overcome childhood adversity and others are not. The most common factor for children who do well despite experiencing adverse events is having a stable, supportive relationship, which helps them respond to adversity in ways which promote recovery. *'Additionally, when caregivers actively help children develop skills to interact with others and to cope with stress, this capacity to manage stress lessens the effect of toxic stress – essentially transforming it to tolerable stress'* (Herndon and Waggoner, 2021: 30). Such secure, stable and nurturing relationships help children thrive, reach their potential and overcome the likelihood of long-term harm linked to ACEs (CDC, 2024). When we prevent or reduce the impact of ACEs, we also prevent potential later involvement in crime, alcohol and substance misuse, depression, self-harm and suicide, alongside reducing risks of long-term ill-health through conditions like cancer, diabetes and heart disease (CDC, 2024). Resilience can best be established by providing safe environments, giving attention where it is needed, building trust in relationships, listening to feelings when these are expressed and providing opportunities for success (Pizzolongo and Hunter, 2011).

Actions health practitioners can take

- Talk with children about their mental health and hold supportive conversations around any challenges they are experiencing.
- Help children and young people learn how to recognise and manage emotions by positively supporting the expression of feelings.
- Keep an eye out for any unusual or exaggerated signs of stress and distress such as social withdrawal, changes in school performance, anger and altered patterns of eating and sleeping.
- Guide parents in positively reinforcing their children through praise, as this plays a key role in emotional development and building self-esteem.
- Support parents and families with understanding and actioning the above.

Actions for more widespread change

- Campaign for government policies and adopt organisational policies that provide families with support with childcare costs and healthy nutrition.
- Advocate for workplaces to adopt policies that help parents balance work and family responsibilities like paid time off for caregiving and flexible work schedules.
- Increase opportunities for all families to access quality childcare and education.

- Advocate for government funding to provide free or low-cost, evidence-based training, aimed at enabling schools, community groups and parents to play a substantial part in reducing the impact of ACEs by supporting children's resilience.

Summary of learning points

This chapter has explored a range of theoretical and practical approaches to understanding trauma and supporting people who have experienced trauma. These include:

- The causes of trauma as embedded in attachment and unreliable support systems in the early years of life, affecting brain and psychological development including the ability to form trusting relationships.
- A recognition of the long-term damaging effects of sustained complex trauma caused by physical, psychological, emotional or sexual abuse, as well as through physical and emotional neglect of young people, alongside single-event traumas which may occur at any stage of life.
- The compounding and exacerbating effect of wider societal patterns of inequality and disadvantage, including racism and poverty, which contribute to the lasting effects of traumatic experiences across the lifespan.
- Recognition of the importance of not shaming any individual, and of the key part that health practitioners can play in supporting people to share their stories and take steps towards recovery.

Questions for reflection and discussion

1. What insights have you gained by reading this chapter? How can these insights change the way you work with people who may have experienced trauma?

2. How might you, within your current or any future health and care roles, introduce ways of identifying whether past trauma is impacting on the present actions of patients and service users?
3. Identify ways in which the organisation for which you work can take action to build resilience amongst children and adults who may have experienced either single-event or sustained trauma.
4. In what ways might understanding the impact of trauma on long-term physical and psychological health, support your care planning with all individuals, whether or not you have ascertained that they have experienced trauma?
5. How might identifying past traumas help you in supporting the physical wellbeing of your patients and service users?

Recommended follow-up reading

Bowlby, J. (2005). *A secure base: Clinical applications of attachment theory* (Routledge Classics). Abingdon: Routledge.

Clark, C. and Aboueissa, A. (2021). Nursing students' adverse childhood experience scores: A national survey. *International Journal of Nursing Education Scholarship*, 18(1): 20210013.

Conti-O'Hare, M. (2002). *The nurse as wounded healer: From trauma to transcendence*. Burlington: Jones and Bartlett Learning.

McGarvie, S. (2024). *Attachment theory, Bowlby's stages & attachment styles*. https://positivepsychology.com/attachment-theory/ [Accessed 13th June 2025].

Van der Kolk, B. (2014). *The body keeps the score. Mind, brain and body in the transformation of trauma*. London: Penguin.

References

Alcohol Change. (2018). *The alcohol change report*. https://alcoholchange.org.uk/about-us/the-alcohol-change-report [Accessed 13th June 2025].

Andersen, S.L. (2003, January 1). Trajectories of brain development: Point of vulnerability or window of opportunity? *Neuroscience and Biobehavioral Reviews*, 27(1–2): 3–18.

APA (American Psychiatric Association). (2022). *Diagnostic and statistical manual of mental disorders* (5th ed., text rev.) (DSM-5-TR). https://doi.org/10.1176/appi.books.9780890425787

Bjorklund, D.F. (2022). Human evolution and the neotenous infant. In: Hart, S.L. and Bjorklund, D.F. (eds) *Evolutionary perspectives on infancy. Evolutionary psychology*. Cham: Springer.

Bowlby, J. (1969/1982). *Attachment and loss: Vol. 1. Attachment*. New York: Basic Books.

Bradshaw, J. (2023). *Poverty in the UK and other countries*. cpag.org.uk/sites/default/files/2024-01/CPAG-Poverty-176-poverty-in-the-uk-and-other-countries [Accessed 25th June 2025].

Budiarto, Y. and Helmi, A.F. (2021). Shame and self-esteem: A meta-analysis. *European Journal of Psychology*, 17(2): 131–145.

Carvalho Silva, R., Oliva, F., Barlati, S., Perusi, G., Meattini, M., Dashi, E., Colombi, N., Vaona, A., Carletto, S. and Minelli, A. (2024). Childhood neglect, the neglected trauma. A systematic review and meta-analysis of its prevalence in psychiatric disorders. *Psychiatry Research*, 335: 1–18

CDC (Centers for Disease Control and Prevention). (2024). *Preventing adverse childhood experiences*. Atlanta, GA: National Center for Injury Prevention and Control, Centers for Disease Control and Prevention. https://www.cdc.gov/aces/prevention/index.html [Accessed 13th June 2025].

Dalvie, S. and Daskalakis, N.P. (2021). The biological effects of trauma. *Complex Psychiatry*, 7(1–2): 16–18.

Dunn, E.C., Nishimi, K., Gomez, S.H., Powers, A. and Bradley, B. (2018). Developmental timing of trauma exposure and emotion dysregulation in adulthood: Are there sensitive periods when trauma is most harmful? *Journal of Affective Disorders*, 227: 869–877.

Essex, R., Markowski, M. and Miller, D. (2022). Structural injustice and dismantling racism in health and healthcare. *Nursing Inquiry*, 29: e12441.

Felitti, V.J., Anda, R.F., Nordenberg, D., Williamson, D.F., Spitz, A.M., Edwards, V., Koss, M.P. and Marks, J.S. (1998). Relationship of childhood abuse and household dysfunction to many of the leading causes of death in adults. The adverse childhood experiences (ACE) study. *American Journal of Preventive Medicine*, 14(4): 245–258.

Finkelhor, D., Shattuck, A., Turner, H. and Hamby, S. (2015). A revised inventory of adverse childhood experiences. *Child Abuse & Neglect*, 48: 13–21.

Galatzer-Levy, I.R., Huang, S.H. and Bonanno, G.A. (2018). Trajectories of resilience and dysfunction following potential trauma: A review and statistical evaluation. *Clinical Psychology Review*, 63: 41–55.

George, C. (2025). Attachment, shame, and trauma. *Brain Sciences*, 15: 1–20.

Greenman, P.S., Renzi, A., Monaco, S., Luciani, F. and Di Trani, M. (2024). How does trauma make you sick? The role of attachment in explaining somatic symptoms of survivors of childhood trauma. *Healthcare*, 12(2): 203.

Hamed, S., Bradby, H., Ahlberg, B.M. and Thapar-Björkert, S. (2022). Racism in healthcare: A scoping review. *BMC Public Health*, 22(1): 1–22.

Herndon, M. and Waggoner, C. (2021). Building resilience: Reducing the impact of adverse childhood experiences. *Dimensions of Early Childhood*, 49(1): 28–33.

Hoeboer, C., De Roos, C., van Son, G.E., Spinhoven, P. and Elzinga, B. (2021). The effect of parental emotional abuse on the severity and treatment of PTSD symptoms in children and adolescents. *Child Abuse & Neglect*, 111: 104775.

Hogg, B., Gardoki-Souto, I., Valiente-Gómez, A., Rosa, A.R., Fortea, L., Radua, J., Amann, B.L. and Moreno-Alcázar, A. (2023). Psychological trauma as a trans-diagnostic risk factor for mental disorder: An umbrella meta-analysis. *European Archives of Psychiatry and Clinical Neuroscience*, 273(2): 397–410.

House of Lords, UK Parliament. (2024). *Child poverty: Statistics, causes and the UK's policy response*. https://lordslibrary.parliament.uk/child-poverty-statistics-causes-and-the-uks-policy-response/ [Accessed 13th June 2025].

Humphreys, K.L., LeMoult, J., Wear, J.G., Piersiak, H.A., Lee, A. and Gotlib, I.H. (2020). Child maltreatment and depression: A meta-analysis of studies using the childhood trauma questionnaire. *Child Abuse & Neglect*, 102: 104361.

Jadhakhan, F., Blakemore, A., Guthrie, E., Romeu, D. and Lindner, O. (2022). Prevalence of medically unexplained symptoms in adults who are high users of healthcare services and magnitude of associated costs: A systematic review. *BMJ Open*, 12(10): 1–12

Kelly-Irving, M. and Delpierre, C. (2019). A critique of the adverse childhood experiences framework in epidemiology and public health: Uses and misuses. *Social Policy and Society*, 18(3): 445–456.

Kirkinis, K., Pieterse, A.L., Martin, C., Agiliga, A. and Brownell, A. (2018). Racism, racial discrimination, and trauma: A systematic review of the social science literature. *Ethnicity & Health*, 26(3): 392–412.

Kratzer, L., Knefel, M., Haselgruber, A., Heinz, P., Schennach, R. and Karatzias, T. (2022). Co-occurrence of severe PTSD, somatic symptoms and dissociation in a large sample of childhood trauma inpatients: A network analysis. *European Archives of Psychiatry & Clinical Neuroscience*, 272(5): 897–908.

Lucre, K., Ashworth, F., Copello, A., Jones, C. and Gilbert, P. (2024). Compassion focused group psychotherapy for attachment and relational trauma: Engaging people with a diagnosis of personality disorder. *Psychology and Psychotherapy: Theory, Research and Practice*, 97(2): 318–338.

Lyons-Ruth, K., Li, F.H., Khoury, J.E., Ahtam, B., Sisitsky, M., Ou, Y., Enlow, M.B. and Grant, E. (2023). Maternal childhood abuse versus neglect associated with differential patterns of infant brain development. *Research on Child and Adolescent Psychopathology*, 51(12): 1919–1932.

Maniglio, R. (2009). The impact of child sexual abuse on health: A systematic review of reviews. *Clinical Psychology Review*, 29(7): 647–657.

Marmot, M., Allen, J., Boyce, T., Goldblatt, P. and Morrison, J. (2020). *Health equity in England: The marmot review 10 years on*. Institute of Health Equity. https://www.health.org.uk/reports-and-analysis/reports/health-equity-in-england-the-marmot-review-10-years-on-0 [Accessed 25th June 2025].

McEwen, B.S. (2019). Neurobiological and systemic effects of chronic stress. *Iranian Journal of Gastroenterology & Hepatology (GOVARESH)*, 24(2): 14–23.

McLaughlin, K.A., Weissman, D. and Bitrán, D. (2019). Childhood adversity and neural development: A systematic review. *Annual Review of Developmental Psychology*, 1(1): 277–312.

Melamed, D.M., Botting, J., Lofthouse, K., Pass, L. and Meiser-Stedman, R. (2024). The relationship between negative self-concept, trauma, and maltreatment in children and adolescents: A meta-analysis. *Clinical Child and Family Psychology Review*, 27: 220–234.

Miller, N., Nair, S. and Majumder, P. (2023). Is it "just" trauma? Use of trauma-informed approaches and multi-agency consultation in mental healthcare of looked after children. *BJPsych Bulletin*, 47(6): 337–34.

National Child Traumatic Stress Network. (2020). *About childhood trauma*. National Center for Child Traumatic Stress. https://www.nctsn.org/what-is-child-trauma/about-child-trauma [Accessed 13th June 2025].

National Police Chiefs' Council. (2024). *Violence against women and girls (VAWG)*. National Policing Statement. https://news.npcc.police.uk/resources/vteb9-ec4cx-7xgru-wufru-5vvo6 [Accessed 15th June 2025].

Nelson, J., Klumparendt, A., Doebler, P. and Ehring, T. (2017). Childhood maltreatment and characteristics of adult depression: Meta-analysis. *The British Journal of Psychiatry*, 210(2): 96–104.

NSPCC. (2024a). *Statistics briefing: Children in care*. https://learning.nspcc.org.uk/research-resources/statistics-briefings/looked-after-children [Accessed 13th June 2025].

NSPCC. (2024b). *News: More than 70,000 children in England have a parent struggling with alcohol misuse*. https://www.nspcc.org.uk/about-us/news-opinion/2024/more-than-70000-children-in-england-have-a-parent-struggling-with-alcohol-misuse/ [Accessed 13th June 2025].

Office for National Statistics. (2020). *Child abuse in England and Wales: March 2020*. https://www.ons.gov.uk/peoplepopulationandcommunity/crimeandjustice/bulletins/childabuseinenglandandwales/march2020 [Accessed 13th June 2025].

Olff, M., Hein, I., Amstadter, A.B., Armour, C., Skogbrott Birkeland, M., Bui, E., Cloitre, M., Ehlers, A., Ford, J.D., Greene, T., Hansen, M., Harnett, N.G., Kaminer, D., Lewis, C., Minelli, A., Niles, B., Nugent, N.R., Roberts, N., Price, M., Reffi, A.N., Seedat, S., Seligowski, A.V. and Vujanovic, A.A. (2025). The impact of trauma and how to intervene: A narrative review of psychotraumatology over the past 15 years. *European Journal of Psychotraumatology*, 16(1): 2458406.

Oral, R., Ramirez, M., Coohey, C., Nakada, S., Walz, A., Kuntz, A., Benoit, J. and Peek-Asa, C. (2016). Adverse childhood experiences and trauma informed care: The future of health care. *Pediatric Research*, 79(1): 227–233.

Pizzolongo, P.J. and Hunter, A. (2011). I am safe and secure: Promoting resilience in young children. *YC Young Children*, 66(2): 67–69.

Prior, V. and Glaser, D. (2006). *Understanding attachment and attachment disorders: Theory, evidence and practice*. London: Jessica Kingsley.

Rosenberg, K.R. (2021). The evolution of human infancy: Why it helps to be helpless. *Annual Review of Anthropology*, 50(1): 423–440.

Sachs-Ericsson, N.J., Rushing, N.C., Stanley, I.H. and Sheffler, J. (2016). In my end is my beginning: Developmental trajectories of adverse childhood experiences to late-life suicide. *Aging & Mental Health*, 20(2): 139–165.

Selwyn, C.N., Lathan, E.C., Richie, F., Gigler, M.E. and Langhinrichsen-Rohling, J. (2021). Bitten by the system that cared for them: Towards a trauma-informed understanding of Patients' healthcare engagement. *Journal of Trauma & Dissociation*, 22(5): 636–652.

Shaw, J.A. (2000). Children, adolescents and trauma. *Psychiatric Quarterly*, 71: 227–243.

Shonkoff, J.P., Garner, A.S. and Committee on Psychosocial Aspects of Child and Family Health, Committee on Early Childhood, Adoption, and Dependent Care, &

Section on Developmental and Behavioral Pediatrics. (2012). The lifelong effects of early childhood adversity and toxic stress. *Pediatrics*, 129(1): e232–e246.

Siegel, D.J. (2006). An interpersonal neurobiology approach to psychotherapy. *Psychiatric Annals; Thorofare*, 36,4: 248–256.

Spinazzola, J., van der Kolk, B. and Ford, J.D. (2021). Developmental trauma disorder: A legacy of attachment trauma in victimized children. *Journal Of Traumatic Stress*, 34: 711–720.

Tomoda, A., Nishitani, S., Takiguchi, S., Fujisawa, T.X., Sugiyama, T. and Teicher, M.H. (2024). The neurobiological effects of childhood maltreatment on brain structure, function, and attachment. *European Archives of Psychiatry and Clinical Neuroscience*. 1–20.

Vygotsky, L.S. (1978). *Mind in society: Development of higher psychological processes*. Cambridge, MA: Harvard University Press.

Winnicott, D.W. (2000). *The child, the family, and the outside world*. London: Penguin.

Winston, R. and Chicot, R. (2016). The importance of early bonding on the long-term mental health and resilience of children. *London Journal of Primary Care*, 8(1): 12–14.

Wolff, N. and Shi, J. (2012). Childhood and adult trauma experiences of incarcerated persons and their relationship to adult behavioral health problems and treatment. *International Journal of Environmental Research and Public Health*, 9(5): 1908–1926.

World Health Organisation and United Nations; Office of the High Commissioner for Human Rights. (2023). *Mental health, human rights and legislation: Guidance and practice*, WHO Reference Number: HR/PUB/23/3 (OHCHR).

3

The impact of adverse childhood experiences across the lifespan

Rebecca Turner

Case study

Jimmy's story

I was in my thirties when I first heard the term 'adverse childhood experiences', but although that was the first time I'd heard this label applied to some of the things that happened in my childhood, by that time, I was certainly no stranger to adversity. It was a nurse on an acute mental health ward who asked me whether I had heard about ACEs. He was trying to help me understand that things I'd experienced in my early life were contributing to health problems I was experiencing at that time. I'm not sure whether he realised what a profound impact that conversation had on me, nor the number of burning questions I was left with, as well as a sense of concern about my own past, present and future.

I don't remember Dad ever living at home with us, but I gradually became aware that he had another family who he spent most of his time with. He rarely came over, and if he did it generally ended badly with him and Mum shouting, fighting and throwing things around. Me and my two brothers lived with my mum who spent time going in and out of psychiatric hospital herself. I'm not sure what she was diagnosed with, but looking back, I can imagine that she would be diagnosed with bipolar disorder today. She

DOI: 10.4324/9781003635604-3

had times of great energy and enthusiasm when she said every-thing was going to be different, better, more enjoyable and that we would make a new start. Those times of high energy were inev-itably followed by longer periods of deep withdrawal and depres-sion. It was during these times that she would sometimes end up in hospital and at least twice I'm aware of, that happened after she had tried to kill herself.

We had an Aunty who came to stay when Mum was in hospital, and she met our physical needs for a meal on the table three times a day and clean clothes to wear for school on a Monday. She never hugged us though or said anything kind to us, and most of the time we had little idea of when Mum would be back, why Dad had left us, or who was going to be caring for us from one week to the next.

We three boys expressed our insecurity by fighting with each other and there were many black eyes, split lips and a broken wrist or two from full on physical fights that took place when we were alone. We seemed to have no way of communicating our feelings with each other apart from fighting.

Looking back, it was clear that Aunty had her own problems. She was a drinker and she didn't always hide that, or even attempt to do so. There was one time a social worker turned up. Aunty was asleep on the floor upstairs after consuming more than her usual amount of afternoon brandy. The social worker knocked at the door and asked to speak with her. My brothers were out with friends, and I knew that I was all that stood between us staying at home and being taken into care. If there was one thing we three were convinced of, it was that being taken into care was probably a much worse fate than staying in our current situation. I managed to bluff the situation somehow, refusing the social worker entry by saying that Aunty was asleep after having a big lunch and wouldn't like to be woken up. Although the social worker was insistent, ten-year-old me was more insistent, and eventually she gave up and went away.

Introduction

Early childhood experiences are increasingly associated with implications for both mental and physical health across the life course (Lacey and Minnis, 2019). Literature identifies that adverse childhood experiences (ACEs) are a significant public health concern (Lynch et al., 2013; Olsen and Warring, 2018) and that the associated costs are substantial (Smith-Battle et al., 2022). Within the United Kingdom, key reports (Cooper and Mackie, 2016; Director of Public Health, 2018; Marmot et al., 2020) have highlighted the prevalence of ACEs and acknowledge the necessity of 'ACE awareness' particularly for the frontline workforce (Riley et al., 2019).

Chapter aims

This chapter develops the exploration of information and ideas around adverse childhood experiences (ACEs) in more detail. The focus of this chapter is:

- What ACEs are.
- The ways in which ACEs affect brain development, attachment and health.
- The prevalence of ACEs in the United Kingdom and further afield.
- Patients' lived experiences and the impact of these on their interactions with healthcare staff.

What are ACEs?

The term 'adverse childhood experiences' (ACEs) was developed in the United States following the landmark Kaiser Permanente ACE study (Felitti et al., 1998). ACEs have been described as stressful events that can occur during childhood and that can have implications upon both mental and physical health across the life course (Lacey and Minnis, 2019). Further studies have concluded that ACEs are intra-familial events or conditions resulting in chronic stress responses in the child's immediate environment (Kelly-Irving et al., 2013).

ACEs include physical, emotional, or sexual abuse, witnessing domestic violence, child neglect and growing up in a household with substance misuse, mental illness, parental separation or divorce, or incarceration of a member of the household (Jones et al., 2019). Current opinion identifies further adversities or negative circumstances that can occur during childhood, which are associated with poor adult outcomes, such as community violence, discrimination, peer victimisation, low birthweight, child disability and economic disadvantage (Asmussen et al., 2020).

This is further acknowledged by Marmot et al. (2020) who identified that children and young people living in deprived areas and in poverty are more likely to be exposed to ACEs when compared to more economically advantaged peers. ACEs can occur most frequently when families are living in highly stressful circumstances, which include low family income and high levels of community deprivation, with adults living in the most deprived quintile being three times more likely to report four or more ACEs in comparison with those living in the least deprived quintile (Bellis et al., 2013). Social inequalities not only increase the likelihood of childhood adversity but can also elevate their negative impact (Asmussen et al., 2020). Indeed, traumatic experiences are known to increase the risk of changes in brain development of children, with negative experiences and insufficient stimulation having an adverse impact on the brain structures and neural connections that form the basis for cognitive and social development (Moody, 2023). Consequently, such neurological changes increase the risk of health, behavioural and social outcomes that can affect individuals in childhood and throughout the life course (Felitti et al., 1998). Additionally, chronic stress in early life alters the development of neurological, hormonal and immunological systems leading to individuals' body systems being locked into a higher state of alertness. In response to such physiological changes, an increased risk of premature ill-health occurs, due to an increased predisposition to developing cancer and heart disease (Public Health Wales, 2015). The body of evidence suggests that ACEs are a significant public health concern (Lynch et al., 2013) and that these experiences in childhood are likely to result in poor health outcomes throughout adult life (Asmundson and Afifi, 2020).

The concept of ACEs has been globally recognised following Felitti et al.'s (1998) landmark study in the United States of America. The momentum continued in America with further research conducted by Nadine Burk and her colleagues (Burke et al., 2011). She identified the relationship between experiencing childhood trauma and poor adult health outcomes. Within the United Kingdom, Public Health Wales contributed to a growing awareness of ACEs through the publication of reports illustrating the prevalence of ACEs in England and Wales (for example, Riley et al., 2019). The term 'ACE Aware' has been further championed and gained momentum through research conducted by Mark Bellis and colleagues (2013), while the Welsh government has offered specific training to frontline workers, such as health visitors and the police (Riley et al., 2019). Similarly, the NHS in Scotland has recognised childhood trauma and the correlation with poor physical and mental health outcomes across the life course as a priority for intervention. The Scottish Health Network (Cooper and Mackie, 2016) presented a case for preventative action on childhood adversity. This report supported the Scottish government's national approach to 'Getting It Right for Every Child' (GIRFEC) (Coles et al., 2016). A further report by the Director of Public Health (2018) identified the term 'ACE Awareness' and instigated the concept of a trauma-informed approach to healthcare within Scotland. In England, the Department for Health and Social Care has developed trauma-informed training materials although this notion of providing training in being trauma-informed appears less developed (Asmussen et al., 2020).

The impact of ACEs

Brain development and attachment

Human brain development is a complex process, with formation of the brain starting several weeks after conception (Waite and Ryan, 2020). The brain is not mature at birth, and brain development is not thought to be complete until the age of around 25 years (Obadina, 2013). Within the first 3 years of life, the most robust growth takes place. From the age of 2 years, the neural connections within the brain are strengthened if used, and discarded if not (Waite and Ryan, 2020). During puberty, there is more growth within the higher cortical regions that involve planning, impulse control, reasoning and self-regulation (Obadina, 2013).

A child's environment and relationships with the primary caregiver play a vital role in the development of the brain and attachment. Attachment theory originates from the work of Bowlby (1969/1982), who asserted that children must feel safe, secure, nurtured and protected. Being neglected or rejected may disrupt a child's psychological development. Furthermore, Waite and Ryan (2020) identified that child separation due to parental incarceration results in insecure attachment due to the physical separation caused by parental imprisonment, leading to disrupted attachment bonds.

Impact on health

Within paediatrics, research suggests associations between ACEs and the following health outcomes: impaired growth and cognitive development, higher risks for childhood obesity, asthma, infections, non-febrile illnesses and disordered sleep (Lopez et al., 2020). These outcomes are, however, dependent upon the age at which ACEs occur and the specific type of exposure. In their systematic review of research literature, Lopez et al. (2020) found an association between parental violence and obesity in childhood, while sexual abuse was associated with youth obesity. Evidence suggests that for each additional ACE, children are 29–44% more likely to have complex health problems with additional health needs across the domains of development, physical health and mental wellbeing (Brown et al., 2019). ACEs are therefore a significant public health concern, which can affect the health and wellbeing of children and young people not just at the time when ACEs occur, but across the entire lifespan (Kalmakis and Chandler, 2015), increasing the chances of living with illness, disability and social challenges in adulthood, and ultimately leading to an early death.

Studies based on the adult population have associated a correlation with childhood adversity and the incidence of cancer, heart disease, obesity and diabetes in adulthood (Bryan, 2019). In addition, there is a known impact on mental ill-health, including rates of suicide, anxiety, depression and being diagnosed with personality disorders (Scully et al., 2020). Moreover, traumatic exposures that are neglectful, abusive and unpredictable in childhood have been linked to an adjustment of the brain structure. This is supported by Kelly-Irving et al. (2013) who identified alterations in the neurobiological stress–response systems, which have implications for health and emotional wellbeing. Further research acknowledges the association of childhood trauma and the incidence of developing health-harming behaviours such as smoking, alcoholism, substance misuse, a history of sexually transmitted infections and a higher number of sexual partners (Scott, 2021).

Research also acknowledges that exposure to childhood adversity is linked to lower educational attainment, as well as unemployment (Metzler et al.,

2017) and poverty (Marmot et al., 2020). Social inequalities increase the likelihood of ACEs and amplify the negative impact (Asmussen et al., 2020). Marmot et al. (2020) highlighted that the presence of ACEs within society impact upon health inequalities and that living in poverty increases the likelihood of experiencing one or more ACE. This is further supported by the Director of Public Health Annual Report (2018), which states that Scottish children living in lower income households are more than six times as likely to have experienced multiple adversities within childhood by the age of 8, compared to those children living in higher income households. This is further supported by Bellis et al. (2014) who argue that having one ACE increases the likelihood of having additional ACEs, with an ultimate cumulative effect that increases the risk of premature mortality (Hughes et al., 2017).

A range of research literature suggests this cumulative effect of ACEs. Bellis et al. (2013) concluded that ACEs contribute to poor health and social outcomes across the lifespan, resulting in a cyclical effect, where those with higher 'ACE counts' have a higher risk of exposing their own children to ACEs. Studies consistently suggest that child maltreatment and other features of dysfunctional parenting are often shared across generations (Bryan, 2019). Where ACEs are left unaddressed, children and young people remain vulnerable to repeating in adulthood, the learned behaviours associated with the adverse circumstances of childhood, resulting in further dysfunction within the family as the cycle of intergenerational trauma continues (Bryan, 2019).

Nonetheless, not all parents who have experienced ACEs will transmit adversity and trauma to their children, as many actively seek support to break the cycle of adversity they have experienced (Bryan, 2019). Regardless of this, intergenerational trauma is not well understood by all healthcare professionals, which is of concern when it comes to implementing strategies aimed at reducing and managing the impact of ACEs (Olsen and Warring, 2018). This is further supported by Gill et al. (2019) who acknowledge that many health professionals have unmet needs in their in their education and clinical practice, regarding knowledge and understanding of ACEs.

The prevalence of ACEs

A study conducted in Wales in 2015 found that 47% of adults in Wales had experienced one type of adversity during their childhood and 14% had experienced four or more (Public Health Wales, 2015; Riley et al., 2019).

In comparison, a recent survey conducted in California in the United States found that 60% of participants have experienced at least one ACE, while 23% of youth and 30% of parents and caregivers have experienced four or more ACEs (Newsom, 2024). However, Asmussen et al. (2020) argue that current estimates of ACE prevalence are imprecise because it can be difficult for adults to recall ACEs. Equally, child abuse and child neglect will often be unreported (Waite and Ryan, 2020). Similarly, Lopez et al. (2020) acknowledge that preschool children are at greatest risk of child abuse and neglect but may be unable to report these experiences due to their limited vocabulary. Moreover, people of all ages may be reluctant to disclose experiences of childhood adversity due to feelings of shame and stigma. Furthermore, studies are unlikely to include people who have died at an early age (Director of Public Health, 2018).

When reviewing the prevalence of ACEs within the healthcare worker population, Maunder et al. (2010) reported that ACEs among healthcare workers is no lower than in the community. Moreover, they identified a correlation between individuals who have experienced adversity as a child and having a desire to seek opportunities to work in a caring profession as an adult. This is supported by Mercer et al. (2023) who, in a systematic review of research literature, found that ACEs were frequently reported and occurred more often among health and social care workers than in the general population.

Lived experience of ACEs and interactions with the healthcare team

Current practice within the United Kingdom does not advocate screening for ACEs. However, it has been recognised that screening young people for ACEs and offering appropriate interventions are key to buffering the impact of such experiences and could reduce the association of poor health outcomes across the life course (Choi et al., 2023).

Research considering ACEs and the use of health and care services within the United Kingdom is scarce. However, a pilot study by Ford et al. (2024) found that individuals with four or more ACEs were more likely to perceive that healthcare professionals do not care about their health. Also, individuals exposed to multiple ACEs were more likely to report poor childhood experiences with healthcare providers. This association between ACEs and experiences in the use of healthcare suggests that improving such relationships (for example, through increasing our knowledge and awareness of trauma) may help to increase trust in healthcare professionals (Ford et al., 2024).

Childhood trauma and interaction with healthcare professionals in clinical practice is thought to trigger a maladaptive stress response (Valeras et al., 2019) and can affect emotional regulation (Ford et al., 2024). Medical and nursing interventions, which involve exposure of body parts, physical touch and invasive procedures, may trigger memories of childhood trauma (Williams, 2023). Therefore, healthcare professionals should consider embedding a trauma-informed approach in the delivery of all health and care services. Similarly, Baca and Salsbury (2023) acknowledge the creation and maintenance of a safe and trusting environment as an important element of trauma informed care, while Valeras et al. (2019) conclude that a more trusting patient and healthcare professional relationship enhances trauma-informed practice within a clinical setting.

Trust and safety were identified by Sodal et al. (2023) as key factors in situations where people are asked to disclose ACEs. Unsurprisingly, they found that the disclosure of ACEs is distressing, making it unlikely that people will disclose these experiences unless they feel comfortable doing so. It has also been argued that people who have lived experience of ACEs can be reluctant to disclose this information due to feeling shame and guilt about their experiences (Larkin and Cairns, 2020). This is further supported by Ford et al. (2024) who identified that people who have experienced four or more ACEs were more than twice as likely to report low levels of comfort in using healthcare services. Therefore, a more trauma-informed approach in clinical settings may help those people who have previously experienced childhood trauma to feel more comfortable in using services and in discussing their healthcare needs.

Tools for now: small changes that can make a big difference

As healthcare practitioners, we can work to:

1. Provide cross-generational support to children and their parents, carers and families as well as to other adults affected by ACEs, with a view to reducing and preventing psychological trauma resulting from adversity.

2. Develop trauma-informed and trauma-responsive workforces and services (see Chapter 8).
3. Raise awareness amongst children, young people, schools, families and community groups about the effects of trauma and adversity.
4. Create a psychologically safe environment for disclosure for children and adults.
5. Protect children and young people from harm through effective approaches to safeguarding and appropriate follow-up.
6. Empower patients and service users, supporting them to talk about their experiences and recognising that what has happened to them can be a more influential aspect in their long-term wellbeing, than diagnostic labelling.
7. Recognise that what you can do in your everyday practice is limited and that taking a supportive approach to signposting to other services might be the most effective way of providing support.

Reducing the impact of ACEs: systemic and longer-term approaches

The importance of positive relationships to support healthy child development is well recognised in research, which suggests that when children have a safe and nurturing environment and positive relationships with parents or carers, they will be likely to experience healthy development. Moreover, when a child or young person has a trusted adult in their life, this has been identified as protecting children from the impact of childhood adversity (Frederick et al., 2023). The following three interventions can potentially support change at a societal level:

1. Strengthening families through funded parenting programmes and family education, using a trauma-informed approach that enables parents to make sense of their past and the present, along with the multifaceted aspects of their own experiences, which can fuel unhelpful actions with their own children.
2. An essential aspect of this wider provision is to offer specialist attachment-focused parenting programmes providing support to parents who have a complex history of childhood trauma. Research acknowledges that protective factors and family strengths are important to develop when

implementing interventions that promote resilience among children of parents or carers with a history of childhood adversity (Woods-Jaeger et al., 2018). However, Asmussen et al. (2020) identified that although protective factors have been found to increase resilience, the specific processes that promote resilience are not yet clearly identified within research literature.

3. There is a particular place for children and young people's nurses and allied health professionals working in schools, in the light of the correlation between childhood adversity and risks associated with smoking, alcohol misuse and illicit drug use during adolescence. Social processes that contribute to health-harming behaviours could be reduced or stopped through school-based interventions aimed at discouraging children and young people from using harmful substances. In turn, some health practitioners are well placed in terms of their knowledge and training, to offer support with alternative coping strategies (Asmussen et al., 2020).

Summary of learning points

Within this chapter:

- ACEs have been described as stressful events that can occur during childhood and across the life course that can have implications for development and for mental and physical health.
- ACEs have been identified as a significant public health concern, which can affect the health and wellbeing of children and young people, not just at the time when the ACEs occur, but also across the lifespan.
- Exploration of the association between ACEs and the use of healthcare suggests that improving professionals' knowledge and awareness of trauma may help to increase patients' trust in healthcare professionals.
- ACEs can be prevented by promoting positive relationships between adults and children, strengthening families, building resilience and through school-based interventions.

Questions for reflection and discussion

1. Within the case study, what are the potential short- and longer-term impacts of the ACEs experienced by Jimmy and his brothers?
2. If Jimmy or another member of his family became a patient on your case load, or attended your clinic or ward, what would your priorities be in terms of interventions to prevent damage and promote recovery? Explain your choice of approach.
3. Identify any other professionals with whom it would be helpful to discuss your concerns in order to better support Jimmy and his family.
4. Jimmy suggests a distrust of social workers and expresses concern that their interventions could make things worse. Describe your overall strategy to build a psychologically safe environment of trust where people like Jimmy and his siblings could share their experiences.
5. Is there anything you would avoid doing or saying with the young Jimmy, or with the adult Jimmy, to reduce or prevent the risk of retraumatisation?

Recommended follow-up reading

Burke Harris, N. (2018). *The deepest well: Healing the long-term effects of childhood adversity.* London: Pan Macmillan.

Maunder, R. and Hunter, J. (2021). *Damaged. Childhood trauma, adult illness, and the need for a health care revolution.* Toronto: University of Toronto Press.

Perry, B. and Szalavitz, M. (2017). *The boy who was raised as a dog.* New York: Basic Books.

Pringle, J., Whitehead, R., Milne, D., Scott, E. and McAteer, J. (2018). The relationship between a trusted adult and adolescent outcomes: A protocol of a scoping review. *Systematic Reviews*, 7(1): 1–7.

Waite, R. and Ryan, R. (2020). *Adverse childhood experiences. What students and health professionals need to know.* London: Routledge.

References

Asmundson, G. and Afifi, T. (2020). *Adverse childhood experiences. Using evidence to advance research, practice, policy and prevention*. London: Elsevier.

Asmussen, K., Fischer, F., Drayton, E. and McBride, T. (2020). *Adverse childhood experiences. What we know, what we don't know, and what should happen next*. London: Early Intervention Foundation. https://www.eif.org.uk/report/adverse-childhood-experiences-what-we-know-what-we-dont-know-and-what-should-happen-next [Accessed 13th June 2025].

Baca, K. and Salsbury, S. (2023). Adverse childhood experiences and trauma informed care for chiropractors: A call to awareness and action. *Chiropractic & Manual Therapies*, 31(30): 1–16.

Bellis, M., Hughes, K., Leckenby, N., Hardcastle, K., Perkins, C. and Lowey, H. (2014). Measuring mortality and the burden of adult disease associated with adverse childhood experiences in England: A national survey. *Journal of Public Health*, 37(3): 445–454.

Bellis, M., Lowey, H., Leckenby, N., Hughes, K. and Harrison, D. (2013). Adverse childhood experiences: Retrospective study to determine their impact on adult health behaviours and health outcomes in a UK population. *Journal of Public Health*, 36(1): 81–91.

Bowlby, J. (1969/1982). *Attachment and loss: Vol. 1. Attachment*. New York: Basic Books.

Brown, S.M., Bender, K., Orsi, R., McCrae, J.S., Phillips, J.D. and Rienks, S. (2019). Adverse childhood experiences and their relationship to complex health profiles among child welfare-involved children: A classification and regression tree analysis. *Health Services Research*, 54(4): 902–911.

Bryan, R. (2019). Getting to why: Adverse childhood experiences' impact on adult health. *The Journal for Nurse Practitioners*, 15(2): 153–157.e1.

Burke, N.J., Hellman, J.L., Scott, B.G., Weems, C.F. and Carrion, V.G. (2011). The impact of adverse childhood experiences on an urban pediatric population. *Child Abuse & Neglect: The International Journal*, 35(6): 408–413.

Choi, K., Boudreau, A. and Dunn, E. (2023). Raising the bar for measuring childhood adversity. *The Lancet*, 7: 81–83.

Coles, E., Cheyne, H., Rankin, J. and Daniel, B. (2016). Getting it right for every child: A national policy framework to promote children's well-being in Scotland, United Kingdom. *The Milbank Quarterly*, 94(2): 334–365.

Cooper, S. and Mackie, P. (2016). *'Polishing the diamonds' addressing adverse childhood experiences in Scotland*. Scottish Public Health Network (ScotPHN). www.scotphn.net/wp-content/uploads/2016/06/2016_05_26-ACE-Report-Final-AF.pdf [Accessed 26th June 2025].

Director of Public Health, Annual Report (2018). *Adverse childhood experiences, resilience, and trauma informed care: A public health approach to understanding and responding to adversity*. www.nhshighland.scot.nhs.uk/media/q1ep0mqj/dph_annual_report_2018.pdf [Accessed 13th June 2025].

Felitti, V., Anda, R., Nordenberg, D., Williamson, D., Spitz, A., Edwards, V., Koss, M. and Marks, J. (1998). Relationship of childhood abuse and household dysfunction to many of the leading causes of death in adults. The adverse childhood experiences (ACE) study. *American Journal of Preventative Medicine*, 14(4): 245–258.

Ford, K., Hughes, K., Cresswell, K., Amos, R. and Bellis, M. (2024). *Adverse childhood experiences and engagement with healthcare services. Findings from a survey of adults in Wales and England.* Cardiff: Bangor University, Public Health Wales NHS Trust.

Frederick, J., Spratt, T. and Devaney, J. (2023). Supportive relationships with trusted adults for children and young people who have experienced adversities: Implications for social work service provision. *British Journal of Social Work*, 53(6): 3129–3145.

Gill, E., Zhan, L., Rosenberg, J. and Breckenridge, L. (2019). Integration of adverse childhood experiences across nursing curriculum. *Journal of Professional Nursing*, 35: 1–8.

Hughes, K., Bellis, M., Hardcastle, K., Sethi, D., Butchart, A., Mikton, C., Jones, L. and Dunne, M. (2017). The effect of multiple adverse childhood experiences on health: A systematic review and meta-analysis. *The Lancet*, 2: 356–366.

Jones, C.M., Merrick, M.T. and Houry, D.E. (2019). Identifying and preventing adverse childhood experiences. Implications for clinical practice. *JAMA*, 323(1): 25.

Kalmakis, K.A. and Chandler, G.E. (2015). Health consequences of adverse childhood experiences: A systematic review. *Journal of American Association of Nurse Practitioners*, 27(8): 457–456.

Kelly-Irving, M., Lepage, B., Dedieu, D., Bartley, M., Blane, D., Grosclaude, P., Lang, T. and Delpierre, C. (2013). Adverse childhood experiences and premature all-cause mortality. *European Journal of Epidemiology*, 28: 721–734.

Lacey, R. and Minnis, H. (2019). Practitioner review: Twenty years of research with adverse childhood experience scores – Advantages, disadvantages and applications to practice. *Journal of Child Psychology and Psychiatry*, 61(2): 116–130.

Larkin, W. and Cairns, P. (2020). Addressing adverse childhood experiences: Implications for professional practice. *British Journal of General Practice*, 70(693) 160–161.

Lopez, M., Ruiz, M.O., Rovnaghi, C.R., Tam, G.K.Y., Hiscox, J., Gotlib, I.H., Barr, D., Carrion, V.G. and Anand, K.J.S. (2020). The social ecology of childhood and early life adversity. *International Pediatric Research Foundation*, 89: 353–367.

Lynch, L., Waite, R. and Davey, M. (2013). Adverse childhood experiences and diabetes in adulthood: Support for a collaborative approach to primary care. *Contemporary Family Therapy*, 35: 639–655.

Marmot, M., Allen, J., Boyce, T., Goldblatt, P. and Morrison, J. (2020). *Health equity in England: The marmot review ten years on.* https://www.health.org.uk/publications/reports/the-marmot-review-10-years-on [Accessed 13th June 2025].

Maunder, R., Peladeau, N., Savage, D. and Lancee, W. (2010). The prevalence of childhood adversity among health care workers and its relationship to adult life events, distress and impairment. *Child Abuse and Neglect*, 34: 114–123.

Mercer, L., Cookson, A., Simpson-Adkins, G. and Van Vuuren, J. (2023). Prevalence of adverse childhood experiences and associations with personal and professional factors in health and social care workers: A systematic review. *Psychological Trauma: Theory, Research, Practice, and Policy*, 15(S2): 231–245.

Metzler, M., Merrick, M., Klevens, J., Ports, K. and Ford, D. (2017). Adverse childhood experiences and life opportunities: Shifting the narrative. *Children and Youth Services Review*, 72: 141–149.

Moody, A. (2023). Increasing awareness of adverse childhood experiences in nurse practitioner students. *Journal of the American Association of Nurse Practitioners*, 35(1): 79–85.

Newsom, G. (2024). *Governor Newsom proclaims adverse childhood experiences awareness day 5.11.24.* https://www.gov.ca.gov/2024/05/11/governor-newsom- [Accessed 13th June 2025].

Obadina, S. (2013). Understanding attachment in abuse and neglect: Implications for child development. *British Journal of School Nursing*, 8(6): 290–296.

Olsen, J. and Warring, S. (2018). Interprofessional education on adverse childhood experiences for associate degree nursing students. *Journal of Nursing Education*, 57(2): 101–105.

Public Health Wales (2015). *Adverse childhood experiences and their impact on health-harming behaviours in the Welsh adult population.* Public Health Wales NHS Trust. https://www.audit.wales/sites/default/files/2020-12/ACE_Chronic_Disease_report.pdf [Accessed 13th June 2025].

Riley, G.S., Bailey, J.W., Bright, D. and Davies, A.R. (2019). *Knowledge and awareness Of Adverse Childhood Experiences (ACEs) in the public service workforce in Wales: A national survey.* Cardiff: Public Health Wales NHS Trust. https://phw.nhs.wales/news/new-survey-shows-both-good-welsh-public-sector-awareness-of-adverse-childhood-experiences-aces-and-opportunities-for-improvement/knowledge-and-awareness-of-adverse-childhood-experiences-in-the-public-service-workforce-in-wales/[Accessed 13th June 2025].

Scott, K. (2021). Adverse childhood experiences. *InnovAIT*, 14(1): 6–11.

Scully, C., McLaughlin, J. and Fitzgerald, A. (2020). The relationship between adverse childhood experiences, family functioning and mental health problems among children and adolescents: A systematic review. *Journal of Family Therapy*, 42: 291–316.

Smith-Battle, L., Rariden, C., Cibulka, N. and Loman, D. (2022). Adverse childhood experiences as public health threat. *Advanced Journal of Nursing*, 122(3): 11.

Sodal, E., Huddy, V. and McKenzie, J. (2023). Black people's experience of being asked about adverse childhood experiences in the UK: A qualitative study. *Psychology and Psychotherapy: Theory, Research and Practice*, 96: 902–917.

Valeras, A.B., Cobb, E., Prodger, M., Hochberg, E., Allosso, L. and Vanden Hazel, H. (2019). Addressing adults with adverse childhood experiences requires a team approach. *The International Journal of Psychiatry in Medicine*, 54(4–5): 352–360.

Waite, R. and Ryan, R. (2020). *Adverse childhood experiences. What students and health professionals need to know.* London: Routledge.

Williams, B. (2023). Understanding the effects of adverse childhood experiences on older people. *Nursing Older People*, 35(1): 37–42.

Woods-Jaeger, B.A., Cho, B., Sexton, C.C., Slagel, L. and Goggin, K. (2018). Promoting resilience: Breaking the intergenerational cycle of adverse childhood experiences. *Health Education & Behaviour*, 45(5): 772–780.

Understanding and working with people with post-traumatic stress disorder

4

Hannah Bailey

Case study

Lucy's story

Throughout my pregnancy I struggled with anxiety due to previous losses that made me worry that something was going to happen to my daughter. When she was born, she was perfect. However, she struggled with what I was told was colic, eczema and reflux. She would cry, her skin was so sore, and her reflux rivalled something out of the exorcist film, especially if I laid her down after feeding. My friend suggested she might have something called CMPA, cow's milk protein allergy. I took her to the GP, but was told this wasn't something breastfed babies got, and I was just an anxious first-time mum. Desperate, exhausted and drowning in washing, I carried out research online and discovered that CMPA in breastfed babies is uncommon, but most definitely a thing. I therefore cut milk from my diet. The improvement in my daughter was obvious almost immediately, but things were not perfect, and I realised that she may also be reacting to soya and other produce related to a cow, including beef.

Stopping eating chocolate (which meant the loss of a significant emotional support) and the overwhelming and intense intrusive thought that I had hurt or poisoned my daughter triggered post-natal depression. I was under the perinatal team, and they

DOI: 10.4324/9781003635604-4

reassured me that all would be fine, and that my daughter was fine. I was suicidal, making plans and gathering resources to attempt to end my life. I was paranoid, I couldn't eat anything that wasn't in a packet that I had opened myself and I was unable to eat anything without checking and rechecking the ingredients. I was triggered every time my daughter was sick, and unable to understand why she continued to react to something every so often when I was being so diligent.

The perinatal team said I had psychosis. They said I had to be assessed and come and stay on the mother and baby unit, or else they would call a Mental Health Act assessment, and I would be detained. I told them I didn't have psychosis and my daughter really did have allergies, but they said this is what someone with psychosis would say. I ended up staying in the mother and baby unit (MBU), then after a few days they relented and said that I didn't have psychosis after all, so I discharged myself and went home.

It was at this point I found out that they had decided that the allergies were a figment of my imagination and that as I had modified my diet and my daughter was still reacting, I must in fact be abusing her and making her sick, so I was referred to Children's Services. I found this out when they contacted me to question me about what I was doing to my daughter.

Not being believed, accusations of psychosis, being put into the MBU, and then being accused of hurting my baby when the entire focus of my mental ill health was being upset because I believed I had hurt my baby, and all the resulting guilt, triggered PTSD. I started experiencing flashbacks, having nightmares and did all I could to avoid professionals and locations that reminded me of my experiences. I continued checking ingredients and being overprotective of my daughter, in case I was accused of hurting her again.

Eventually, I was able to access support from an alternative Trust who helped me process what I had been through by writing scripts about what had happened, and then rewriting them with what I knew at the time, so that the trauma memories were *gradually sorted and filed correctly. My daughter also reached the top of the waiting list for consultation at the hospital, and skin prick testing confirmed the issue all along had been an undetected IgE-mediated egg allergy. Thus, I had objective medical evidence of my innocence, which, alongside the treatment for the PTSD, allowed me to move forward.*

However, trauma, in the form of fear of further accusations of abusing my kids, remains with me to this day. I will never understand how the lack of understanding of my daughter's symptoms in the presence of no other symptoms made them accuse me of being the culprit, but I am forever grateful to 'therapy Dave' who helped me recover.

Introduction

Approximately 70% of people globally will experience traumatic events in their lifetime (Kessler et al., 2017). However, only 3.9% of the world's population develops post-traumatic stress disorder (PTSD), which can occur following a wide range of traumatic experiences (Koenen et al., 2017).

Chapter aims

This chapter focuses on PTSD and includes information and ideas related to:

- Some of the brain changes that might be seen in PTSD.
- The symptoms of PTSD and how these impact on people's ability to live fulfilling lives.
- What we can do in the moment as healthcare professionals to support people living with PTSD and others who have had traumatic experiences.
- Specialist treatments for which people living with PTSD may be referred.

The brain and PTSD

To understand the symptoms of PTSD, it is helpful to have an overview of changes in brain anatomy that are seen following trauma. Central to this are parts of the brain that play roles in memory formation, information processing and emotional regulation. Brain changes in PTSD can be wide-ranging, but this chapter will focus on a few specific areas, rather than considering the whole picture. A key consideration in exploring these changes is that our brain's goal is to keep us safe from danger and that sometimes it goes about this in ways that lead to unhelpful experiences, which become the signs of trauma and the symptoms of PTSD in a person who has experienced trauma. In this chapter, the focus is on those for whom trauma has occurred as a single event or is of a time-limited nature, sometimes associated with the work of uniformed and armed services personnel, road traffic incidents or one-off assaults. The changes seen in the brain following such events need to be understood in relation to the symptoms and difficulties, which then disrupt everyday life for the traumatised person.

The first structure to consider is the thalamus, which receives information from the senses (touch, sight, smell, sound and taste) and then processes this information before sending it onwards to be dealt with by other brain structures. Further research is needed to fully understand the role of the thalamus in PTSD (Yoshii, 2021). However, current knowledge suggests that following exposure to a traumatic event, the thalamus can decline (Kuhn et al., 2021; Yoshii, 2021) and that there is a link between the diminished volume of the thalamus and increased symptoms of PTSD, such as re-experiencing the traumatic event through flashbacks (Yoshii, 2021).

Also thought to contribute to PTSD are the amygdala, which are situated on both the left and right sides of the brain. The amygdala scan information coming from the thalamus and from our thoughts, looking for potential risks and acting as an alarm system. They provide quick bursts of emotion (such as anxiety or anger) to ensure a swift reaction to threats identified by the thalamus (Kredlow et al., 2022). In one analysis, Woon and Hedges (2009) found that the amygdala store emotional memories, where a threat has been experienced or something has occurred from which we need to learn. This particularly applies to memories that are fear-inducing or those with a strong focus on body sensations. An example of this type of memory would be when something is eaten that causes nausea and vomiting. The next time the same food is seen or smelt, feelings of sickness and nausea can also recur, even without eating the food. The amygdala, having learned that the food could be a threat to health, recreate the feelings of sickness, reminding us to avoid the food and keep safe.

People living with PTSD have been shown to have an increase in activity of the amygdala (Nutt and Malizia, 2004; Sherin and Nemeroff, 2011; Woon and Hedges, 2009). This suggests the likelihood of more scanning for threats and dangers, or potentially greater reactivity. Interestingly, in a study of armed forces personnel who had been exposed to trauma but who did not develop PTSD, no significant change was found in the amygdala (Kuhn et al., 2021). However, there is no clear change in the size of the amygdala in people with PTSD compared to control groups (Woon and Hedges, 2009), only in the activity and reactivity.

The hippocampus tries to make sense of and file information coming from the amygdala. If it finds information which clarifies that there is no threat, the hippocampus begins to calm down the brain's automatic protective reaction (Kredlow et al., 2022). However, if it finds a similar memory or experience where there has previously been a threat, it helps to bring about a more intense response, aimed at keeping us out of danger.

Another role of the hippocampus is to give memories a date and time so that we can understand whether something is happening in the past or the present. This is an important consideration in PTSD, where people experiencing flashbacks perceive these to be happening in the present moment, despite the link being to a past memory.

A reduction in the volume of the hippocampus is common in brain scans of people living with PTSD (Nutt and Malizia, 2004; Sherin and Nemeroff, 2011) alongside decreased neuronal connectivity (Kredlow et al., 2022). The hippocampus is involved in helping us unlearn conditioned responses (Kredlow et al., 2022), although a reduction in its ability to do this can mean that we are less able to separate emotions and reactions from the situations that elicit them.

Returning to the example of the food causing sickness – if on a subsequent occasion the food is eaten despite the initial disgust and nausea response, yet this does not lead to an unpleasant reaction, it becomes more likely that the next time the food is seen there will not be the same intensity of disgust. The hippocampus recognises that it is safe and moderates information coming in from the amygdala (Figure 4.1).

The final brain structure to consider is the frontal cortex, which has a role in regulating emotions, planning and considering the consequences of our

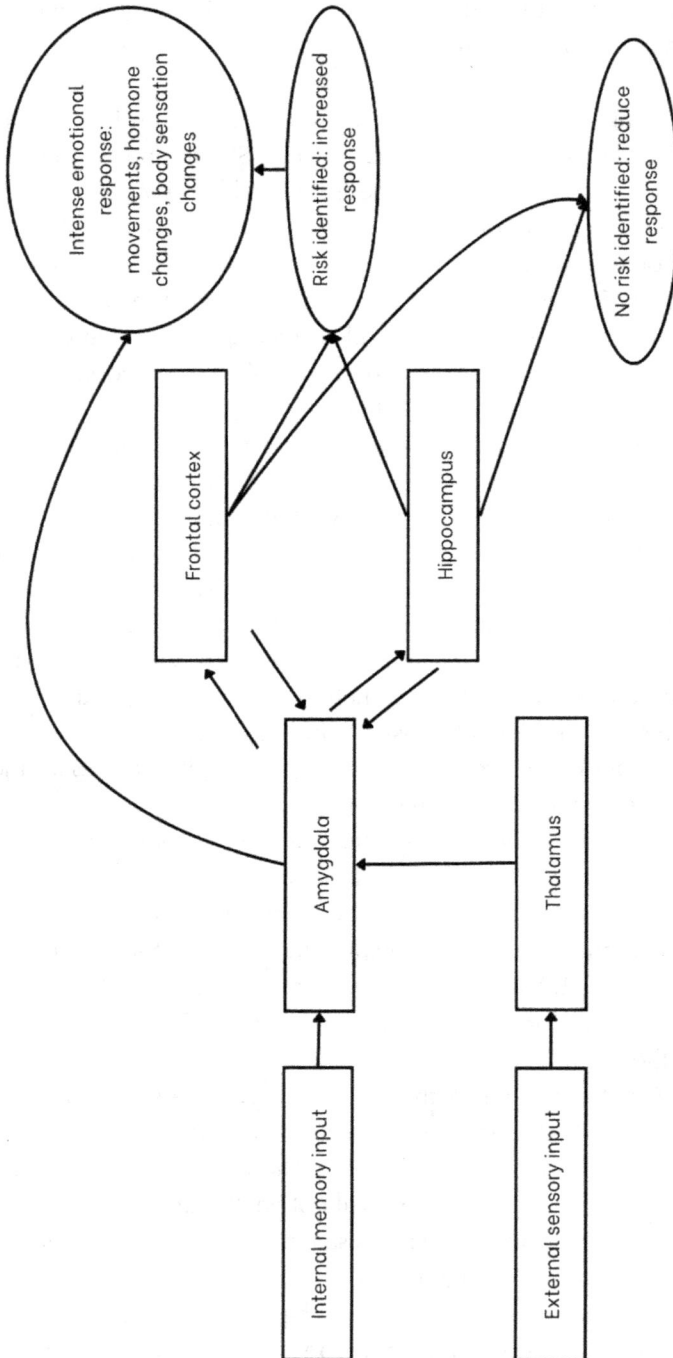

Figure 4.1 Brain areas and structures influencing symptoms of PTSD

actions. It helps us manage the rest of the brain and can contribute to the activation of memories as well as helping to override initial messages coming from the other parts of the brain. The pre-frontal cortex works alongside the hippocampus to reduce our response to threats (Kredlow et al., 2022). For example, it is the part of the brain that might think: *'It is okay to eat this, because I am not sick now'*, so that despite some initial nausea occurring, we are able to reassure ourselves and take appropriate action.

In PTSD, there is some evidence that there is a reduced ability in the pre-frontal cortex to change the experience of the fear response (Nutt and Malizia, 2004; Sherin and Nemeroff, 2011). This makes it harder to unlearn responses to the environment around us. When exposed to stress, even without the development of PTSD, the pre-frontal cortex can become smaller in volume and less connected to other areas of the brain (Kredlow et al., 2022).

It is important to note that research into brain changes has been unable to establish whether changes are due to traumatic experiences or to developing PTSD, or may be a risk factor for developing PTSD. This is because researchers generally only begin scanning individuals' brains after they have had traumatic experiences. Alongside inconsistencies in results, this makes it difficult to demonstrate causation (Kredlow et al., 2022; Kuhn et al., 2021; Sherin and Nemeroff, 2011; Woon and Hedges, 2009). Most studies also have relatively small sample sizes (Kredlow et al., 2022; Woon and Hedges, 2009) and a limited ability to create controls. For example, one hypothesis is that different traumatic experiences elicit different responses and changes in the brain, but it would be difficult to prove this as all traumas are uniquely experienced due to the context provided by previous life events.

Another aspect making brain changes difficult to research is the differences in the period of time individuals have been living with PTSD and variations in the time since the trauma occurred (Woon and Hedges, 2009). Thus, all these changes in the brain present differently with different people, and similarly, there are a broad range of symptoms and behaviours that can be seen in someone living with PTSD.

Symptoms and changes to wellbeing

PTSD has three main groups of symptoms listed in the International Classification of Diseases (ICD-11) (World Health Organisation, 2022) namely re-experiencing, avoidance and persistent perceptions of heightened

Table 4.1 Three groups of PTSD symptoms identified within ICD-11

Re-experiencing	Avoidance	Increased perception of threat
• Vivid thoughts and memories • Nightmares • Flashbacks • Strong overwhelming emotions (such as fear or horror)	• Avoiding activities or situations that are reminders of the event • Avoiding thoughts and memories about the event	• Hypervigilance • Being easily startled, for example by unexpected noises

current threat. For PTSD to be diagnosed, symptoms need to be experienced in a way that limits the person's ability to function in everyday life, for example, participating in work or school. Table 4.1 summarises the symptoms of PTSD as outlined in the ICD-11 (World Health Organisation, 2022).

Re-experiencing

Symptoms of re-experiencing include intense mental and physical experiences that emerge relating to the trauma (Sherin and Nemeroff, 2011) in the form of:

- Flashbacks.
- Intrusive thoughts, including vivid memories and images.
- Nightmares and repetitive dreams.

Lucy, in the case study which began this chapter, describes experiencing flashbacks to her experiences as well as ongoing nightmares. When people with PTSD are reminded of the trauma, they endured they often experience extremely strong emotions, which recreates the distress, fear and horror felt at the time of the event. These emotions can also lead to intense physical sensations (World Health Organisation, 2022). The person may experience these emotions without a strong thought or memory, in response to reminders about the event. This links to the idea of having a physical feeling of sickness when smelling something that previously made us unwell, even in the absence of vivid memories of the earlier episode of vomiting. The brain works to keep us safe from a repeat trauma.

Lucy could conceivably experience a flashback if receiving a telephone call from a health professional, or if her daughter became unwell for any reason, or in hospital environments. This may be in the form of visual flash-backs, as if she is back in hospital herself, or re-experiencing the accusatory telephone calls. Alternatively, it could be in the form of a body memory where she experiences the emotion, perhaps fear or horror, and the intense physical sensations associated with these in her body, without the related memories and images arising. People living with PTSD may use avoidance strategies to reduce the number of flashbacks they experience, in an effort to reduce the likelihood of revisiting the distress.

Avoidance

When experiencing avoidance people seek to reduce the risk of re-exposure (Sherin and Nemeroff, 2011).

- They may deliberately avoid reminders of the traumatic event. This could include avoidance of thoughts or memories or avoidance of people, situations or conversations that remind them of the event. People sometimes describe building a wall around themselves to try and avoid thoughts and emotions, although this is rarely found to be an effective strategy.
- A person may also try to numb themselves, perhaps using drugs or alcohol (World Health Organisation, 2022) or withdraw from things they used to do. Some people experience dissociation, depression or derealisation (Sherin and Nemeroff, 2011).

In this chapter's case study, Lucy mentions avoidance behaviours after her experiences, including avoiding professionals and places that remind her of her trauma. It is possible that she will also have experienced other symptoms associated with avoidance, including depression and social withdrawal. Such symptoms could affect other areas of life, such as Lucy's ability to access healthcare for herself, her ability to work and relationships with friends and family.

People who use avoidance can experience their world becoming smaller as more and more people and situations are avoided to try and manage symptoms. They may struggle to leave their homes, or to access help and attend social events, leading to increasingly limited opportunities for social interaction. They may adopt unhelpful ways of trying to cope and manage in these situations, perhaps using drugs or alcohol to numb emotions or responses they cannot avoid.

Increased perception of threat

In considering the final group of symptoms, persistent perceptions of heightened current threat, it can be helpful to think of these as activating symptoms (Sherin and Nemeroff, 2011). There may be:

- Hypervigilance and hyperarousal.
- Increased startle responses and jumpiness.
- Insomnia.
- Agitation.
- Impulsivity.
- Irritability and anger.

People experiencing these activating symptoms may respond quickly and be hypervigilant. For example, they may react to loud noises or flinch if touched unexpectedly. Often feeling under immediate threat in some situations, they work hard to protect themselves from this. Some of the actions taken in response to the perceived threat include such things as checking locks, having to sit facing an exit or close to a door, restlessness or finding it difficult to remain calm, in addition to irritability when startled or having feelings of being unsafe and out of control.

In the case study, Lucy demonstrates specific types of hypervigilance in the form of checking the ingredients of food and being overprotective of her daughter. While she may have checked the food upon learning of her daughter's allergy anyway, the thoroughness of her checking appears to have increased to such an extent that there were concerns about her potentially having developed psychosis.

It is noteworthy that the ICD-11 (World Health Organisation, 2022) states that symptoms of hypervigilance can appear to be like paranoia but that such symptoms are not evidence of psychosis. Similarly, flashbacks may be misinterpreted by professionals as being hallucinations, due to the intensity of the person's experience of being back in the moment when the trauma occurred. These are not psychotic experiences either (World Health Organisation, 2022).

It is common for people with PTSD to experience a whole range of painful emotions, including anger, shame and guilt. This may include guilt for surviving an event when others did not. Such symptoms have an impact on people's relationships, as well as on their ability to work and function in daily life. Ultimately, such symptoms can also make it difficult to access support from appropriate services.

Co-occurring conditions

Alongside the mental health symptoms of PTSD, there are a wide range of physical health consequences and complications associated with experiencing trauma. Healthcare practitioners need to consider this when offering support and treatment to individuals for any aspect of their health. Considering whether PTSD could be a contributing factor to physical symptoms can be helpful to understanding the person and their presentation (Megnin-Viggars et al., 2019; Sommer et al., 2021).

For people who have experienced trauma, there is a significant increased risk of cardiovascular disease and symptoms, along with metabolic disorders (D'Andrea et al., 2011; Krantz et al., 2022). Changes in the functioning of the immune system have also been observed, with people being more likely to experience irritable bowel syndrome (IBS) and other gastrointestinal disorders such as ulcers, as well as experiencing musculoskeletal problems and pain disorders such as fibromyalgia. Correlations with reproductive disorders and gynaecological disorders for women have also been identified (D'Andrea et al., 2011).

Due to the wide-ranging physiological as well as psychological changes across all body systems, questions are arising about whether PTSD needs to be treated as a systemic, rather than purely psychological disorder (Krantz et al., 2022). Furthermore, given the complexity of the physical health implications, all kinds of healthcare practitioners will encounter people experiencing symptoms of PTSD. Trauma-informed care highlights the importance of understanding this and of assuming that most people, including us and our colleagues, may have experienced a traumatic event at some point in our lives (Emsley et al., 2022). Therefore, all care provision needs to acknowledge that this may impact on every aspect of health, care, communication and social needs.

With this in mind, we will now explore ways in which we can potentially support people who are affected by PTSD.

Tools for now: small changes that can make a big difference

It is important to remember that the people we are meeting in our workplaces may not previously have shared their traumatic experiences with healthcare providers, meaning that they may not have been assessed for

PTSD, and therefore may be experiencing symptoms in the absence of a diagnosis.

Some of the barriers that can prevent people disclosing traumatic experiences are difficult to overcome in the healthcare environment. For example, workers who are rushed will discourage people from disclosing upsetting and traumatic experiences (Jeffreys et al., 2010), regardless of intending to do so. There are also barriers caused by individual communication styles, such as when professionals come across as being distanced, disinterested or judgemental (Jeffreys et al., 2010).

To support individuals to disclose their trauma, professionals need to be hopeful, caring and non-judgemental (Heron and Eisma, 2021; Jeffreys et al., 2010). We need to provide a sense of having time for the person in front of us, paying full attention to the individual in the moment (Jeffreys et al., 2010; Levenson, 2020).

Following a disclosure, it is helpful to provide information about available support alongside reassurance that PTSD is a treatable condition (Jeffreys et al., 2010). While it may sometimes be appropriate to ask directly about whether someone has experienced trauma, as a way of supporting disclosure (Heron and Eisma, 2021; Megnin-Viggars et al., 2019), people should not be asked to describe their trauma experiences in detail. Such in-depth discussions can be psychologically unsafe due to the risk of re-traumatisation (Fisher, 1999).

Some people may want to share details about their experiences so it can be useful to ask individuals whether they feel it would be helpful to share. However, asking whether sharing might cause an increase in symptoms and saying that we do not want to cause any more distress, are also important (Fisher, 1999). This may be challenging where information is needed for assessment, and it is important that, as far as possible, we avoid hurrying people to disclose information, ensuring that a therapeutic alliance is created first (Levenson, 2020).

If aware that someone has a diagnosis or is showing symptoms of PTSD, there are some relatively straightforward techniques, tools and changes that we may be able to put into place. These can support individuals to manage their symptoms, reduce the risk of flashbacks and minimise any distress caused by their treatment.

Helping people regain a sense of control and mastery over their care by involving them in decision making and planning around their treatment can be important (Fletcher et al., 2021; Levenson, 2020). Fletcher et al. (2021)

highlighted that this will involve reflective listening, validation, negotiation and can also require creating a specific plan relating to their PTSD. Even the way we phrase supportive questions can increase a person's sense of control and mastery. For example, rather than saying: *'You look nervous, let's talk'*, it may be more helpful to phrase this as an observation coupled with an opportunity: *'I notice you seem tense at the moment. Would you like to chat about what's happening?'* (Treleaven, 2018).

A number of things could be helpful to include in a care or treatment plan, which should be discussed and then clearly documented for handover to other professionals.

1. Someone's usual sleep hygiene and sleep patterns and trying to replicate these as closely as possible during an in-patient admission as sleep quality impacts on symptom severity (Fletcher et al., 2021).
2. If someone is going to be woken, discuss with them in advance the best way to do this to help reduce the distress this could cause (Fletcher et al., 2021). If they are unsure what may be helpful, just acknowledging that this could be difficult for them is likely to feel validating and supportive.
3. Triggers for flashbacks are different for everyone. Therefore, have conversations about what may trigger flashbacks, and having established what may trigger a flashback, consider ways of reducing exposure to these in that care environment (NICE, 2018). This may include sounds, smells, and specific actions on the part of those working with them, as well as preferences about the gender of workers supporting them.
4. Find out if they have any established strategies for when they are experiencing a flashback or an increase in symptoms and aim to support this practice.

Self-management skills to teach patients and service users

If you are working with someone experiencing symptoms of PTSD, there are some techniques that can be taught quickly to support them to develop self-management skills.

Breathing techniques

Deep breathing and breathing techniques can be useful when people are noticing an increase in their symptoms and can help reduce the intensity of their anxiety or help them ground back to the present moment (Fletcher et al., 2021; Linehan, 2015).

Breathe in - 4 seconds

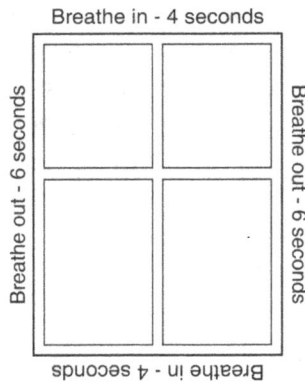

Figure 4.2 Picturing a tall window to support longer outbreaths

You can teach a few different techniques, but paced breathing is often used. This is slowing down the rate of breathing to about 6/7 breaths per minute (Linehan, 2015).

Encourage people to breathe in for 4 seconds and out for 6 seconds. The exact timing is not the focus here as much as attempting to extend the out breath to be longer than the in breath. This starts to downregulate the central nervous system and slow the heart rate (Linehan, 2015). If people find this difficult, begin by encouraging them to count how long they can take an in-breath and try to match their out-breath to this. Some people find it helpful to picture a window or box as they are breathing in and out (Figure 4.2).

Grounding in the present

When we are experiencing intense anxiety, worry or a flashback, we can lose touch with the present moment. The use of grounding techniques can help reduce anxiety by bringing us back to the here and now.

A commonly used technique is the 5, 4, 3, 2, 1 practice. There are various ways this practice is taught but it can be helpful to encourage someone to pay attention to their senses and notice things around them (these need to be things that are not triggering).

- 5 things that they can see, describing these in detail.
- 4 things that they can feel, again describing and noticing in detail (examples include their bottom on the chair, their watch, the coolness of the table under their hand).

- 3 things they can hear, focusing on those sounds.
- 2 things they can smell.
- 1 thing they can taste.

Similarly, some people benefit from looking for specific shapes or colours in the environment, for example, trying to find each colour of the rainbow around them or counting how many circles there are in the room.

The use of a grounding object may be helpful. Some people use sensory 'fidget' toys, while others may prefer something solid such as a pebble that can be carried in the pocket, creating a sense of stability and solidness that they can focus on as they hold it.

Finally, smell is a powerful tool to help with grounding and self-soothing (Fletcher et al., 2021). You could support a person to consider what smells they find soothing or are associated with pleasant memories. It can be helpful to explore whether there is a way they can carry such scents around with them, perhaps considering perfumes, hand creams, or having some sprayed on a tissue (Treleaven, 2018).

Reframing thoughts

Reframing thoughts is a helpful skill for which you may be able to provide support (Kredlow et al., 2022). This can include teaching patients to practice making statements such as:

'I feel frightened, and I am safe now', or

'My name is .... And I am safe right now. It is (day of the week) and the time is ......'.

Making these statements at difficult times, such as when waking from a nightmare, can help with reducing heightened anxiety more swiftly.

Interventions for PTSD: longer-term approaches

Prior to any formal trauma-based therapy being offered by specialist mental health services, the individual must be safe and able to tolerate some of the symptoms they are experiencing (Fisher, 1999; Ford et al., 2005; Zayfert and Black Becker, 2020). This is something that is not always considered by professionals who do not have regular experience in working with individuals living with PTSD.

Specialist services will also consider someone's stability in their symptoms and ability to manage triggers (Fisher, 1999). Initial support is not around processing the trauma but instead focusses on managing symptoms so that these do not interfere with the treatment (Zayfert and Black Becker, 2020). The tools and techniques identified above, which can be taught to service users, are examples of the ways we can help people find stability and navigate their symptoms before progressing to more in-depth therapy.

NICE guidelines (2018) recommend eye movement desensitisation and reprocessing therapy (EMDR) and cognitive behavioural therapy for trauma (TF-CBT). The treatment approach recommended is different depending on the type of trauma and how long symptoms have been occurring. CBT for trauma includes exposure-based approaches to varying degrees (NICE, 2018). Research has found that both EMDR and TF-CBT change connectivity in the brain (Santarnecchi et al., 2019).

TF-CBT combines both exposure and cognitive restructuring (Zayfert and Black Becker, 2020). Exposure involves people facing cues that they may find distressing or challenging. For example, if involved in a car accident and fearful of driving a car, exposure protocols may include spending time as a passenger in a car again, before going on to drive for short journeys whilst being supported to manage the associated anxiety. Cognitive restructuring relates to helping patients change unhelpful or problematic thoughts for thoughts that are more helpful and, importantly, balanced. It is not about always thinking positively (Zayfert and Black Becker, 2020).

EMDR, on the other hand, does not require cognitive restructuring in the same way and instead focuses on exposure to, and the reprocessing of, traumatic memories (Jongh et al., 2024). As previously stated, patients must first learn coping strategies before discussion of and focus on the memory begins. This includes bilateral eye movements, usually guided by a therapist's hand, while the individual is thinking about the memory, though not being encouraged to disclose it to the therapist (Jongh et al., 2024). It is thought that the bilateral movements challenge the patients' working memory while recalling the traumatic event and that this changes how the memory is stored and processed by the brain at the end of the recall period. Ultimately, this leads to a less intensely emotional version of the memory being stored (Jongh et al., 2024; Van den Hout and Engelhard, 2012; Wadji et al., 2022).

Summary of learning points

This chapter has explored the following theoretical and practical approaches to understanding and supporting people living with PTSD:

- Brain changes occur in people who experience a trauma and go on to develop PTSD.
- How trauma and PTSD impact an individual's wellbeing and create symptoms including flashbacks, hypervigilance, and avoidance of triggers that they may live with as a result.
- Health practitioners can help improve experiences of healthcare by focusing on the person, even when in a rushed and busy healthcare environment.
- A range of tools and techniques you can teach people in your care so that they can better support themselves.
- Specialist treatments which are available, including EMDR and trauma-focused CBT.

Questions for reflection and discussion

1. What one thing could you implement, given your current working environment and its limitations, which could support someone living with PTSD who is in your care? Some examples to help generate ideas include the following:
   a. Asking on admission to an in-patient setting about waking preferences. Is this something you could roll out to the MDT to consider supporting sleep hygiene?
   b. Supporting yourself to ground for a moment prior to seeing your patient, perhaps using some of the techniques from this chapter, so you can be more present with them and feel less rushed.
2. How might you word questions to support an increased sense of control? These will depend on the workplace but could include: *'How would you like to be supported with your personal care?*

Is there a time or way you would prefer?' or *'It looks like you are struggling with flashbacks, may I share some tools that could help you?'*

3. Take some time to consider Lucy's case study at the beginning of this chapter. What would you need to put in place or be aware of to support Lucy if she was accessing care in your service? What sort of plan of care would it be useful to outline for Lucy if she was accessing your services?

4. What would you need to understand and what potential triggers or situations could arise that may exacerbate Lucy's PTSD symptoms? What would you want to know and understand more about from her?

5. What barriers may arise for you personally when working with people who have experienced trauma? Are there situations or needs that you have that it is important to be aware of so that you can better support others?

Recommended follow-up reading

Fisher, J. (1999). *The Work of Stabilization in Trauma Treatment.* www. complextrauma.uk/uploads/2/3/9/4/23949705/the_work_on_stabilization_in_trauma_work.pdf

Lee, D. (2012). *Recovering from trauma using compassion focused therapy.* London: Robinson.

The above two texts are included as recommended reading as both contain additional skills and knowledge that we can share with the individuals we are working with. Lee (2012) is a self-help book, which also includes psychoeducation around the brain and development of PTSD. It includes techniques that we can use for ourselves as well as teaching to others. Similarly, Fisher (1999) includes techniques but is written for therapists. Her work includes tools to teach others and the rationale for why further treatments are not offered until patients are stabilised.

References

D'Andrea, W., Sharma, R., Zelechoski, A.D. and Spinazzola, J. (2011). Physical health problems after single trauma exposure: When stress takes root in the body. *Journal of the American Psychiatric Nurses Association*, 17(6): 378–392.

Emsley, E., Smith, J., Martin, D. and Lewis, N.V. (2022). Trauma-informed care in the UK: Where are we? A qualitative study of health policies and professional perspectives. *BMC Health Services Research*, 22: 1164.

Fisher, J. (1999). *The work of stabilization in trauma treatment*. www.complextrauma. uk/uploads/2/3/9/4/23949705/the_work_on_stabilization_in_trauma_work.pdf [Accessed 9th August 2024].

Fletcher, K.E., Steinbach, S., Lewis, F., Hendricks, M. and Kwan, B. (2021). Hospitalized medical patients with posttraumatic stress disorder (PTSD): Review of the literature and a roadmap for improved care. *Journal of Hospital Medicine*, 16(1): 38–43.

Ford, J.D., Courtois, C.A., Steele, K., Hart, O.V.D. and Nijenhuis, E.R. (2005). Treatment of complex posttraumatic self-dysregulation. *Journal of Traumatic Stress: Official Publication of the International Society for Traumatic Stress Studies*, 18(5): 437–447.

Heron, R.L. and Eisma, M.C. (2021). Barriers and facilitators of disclosing domestic violence to the healthcare service: A systematic review of qualitative research. *Health & Social Care in the Community*, 29(3): 612–630.

Jeffreys, M.D., Leibowitz, R.Q., Finley, E. and Arar, N. (2010). Trauma disclosure to health care professionals by veterans: Clinical implications. *Military Medicine*, 175(10): 719–724.

Jongh, A., Roos, C. and El-Leithy, S. (2024). State of the science: Eye movement desensitization and reprocessing (EMDR) therapy. *Journal of Traumatic Stress*, 37: 205–216.

Kessler, R.C., Aguilar-Gaxiola, S., Alonso, J., Benjet, C., Bromet, E.J., Cardoso, G., Degenhardt, L., de Girolamo, G., Dinolova, R.V., Ferry, F. and Florescu, S. (2017). Trauma and PTSD in the WHO world mental health surveys. *European Journal of Psychotraumatology*, 8(5): p1353383.

Koenen, K.C., Ratanatharathorn, A., Ng, L., McLaughlin, K.A., Bromet, E.J., Stein, D.J., Karam, E.G., Ruscio, A.M., Benjet, J., Scott, K., Atwoli, L., Petukhova, M., Lim, C.C.W., Aguilar-Gaxiola, S., Al-Hamzawi, A., Alonso, J., Bunting, B., Ciutan, M., de Girolamo, G., Degenhardt, L., Gureje, O., Haro, J.M., Huang, Y., Kawakami, N., Lee, S., Navarro-Mateu, F., Pennell, B.-E., Piazza, M., Sampson, N., Ten Have, M., Torres, Y., Viana, M.C., Williams, D., Xavier, M. and Kessler, R.C. (2017). Posttraumatic stress disorder in the World Mental Health Surveys. *Psychological Medicine*, 47(13): 2260–2274.

Krantz, D.S., Shank, L.M. and Goodie, J.L. (2022). Post-traumatic stress disorder (PTSD) as a systemic disorder: Pathways to cardiovascular disease. *Health Psychology*, 41(10): 651–662.

Kredlow, M.A., Fenster, R.J., Laurent, E.S., Ressler, K.J. and Phelps, E.A. (2022). Prefrontal cortex, amygdala, and threat processing: Implications for PTSD. *Neuropsychopharmacology*, 47(1): 247–259.

Kuhn, S., Butler, O., Willmund, G., Wesemann, U., Zimmermann, P. and Gallinat, J. (2021). The brain at war: Effects of stress on brain structure in soldiers deployed to a war zone. *Translational Psychiatry*, 11: 247.

Levenson, J. (2020). Translating trauma-informed principles into social work practice. *Social Work*, 65(3): 288–298.

Linehan, M. (2015). *DBT: Skills training manual*. New York: Guilford Press.

Megnin-Viggars, O., Mavranezouli, I., Greenberg, N., Hajioff, S. and Leach, J. (2019). Post-traumatic stress disorder: What does NICE guidance mean for primary care? *British Journal of General Practice*, 69(684): 328–329.

NICE (2018). *Post-traumatic stress disorder*. www.nice.org.uk/guidance/ng116 [Accessed 9th August 2024].

Nutt, D.J. and Malizia, A.L. (2004). Structural and functional brain changes in post-traumatic stress disorder. *Journal of Clinical Psychiatry*, 65: 11–17.

Santarnecchi, E., Bossini, L., Vatti, G., Fagiolini, A., La Porta, P., Di Lorenzo, G., Siracusano, A., Rossi, S. and Rossi, A. (2019). Psychological and brain connectivity changes following trauma-focused CBT and EMDR treatment in single-episode PTSD patients. *Frontiers in Psychology*, 10: 129.

Sherin, J.E. and Nemeroff, C.B. (2011). Post-traumatic stress disorder: The neurobiological impact of psychological trauma. *Dialogues in Clinical Neuroscience*, 13(3): 263–278.

Sommer, J.L., Reynolds, K., El-Gabalawy, R., Pietrzak, R.H., Mackenzie, C.S., Ceccarelli, L., Mota, N. and Sareen, J. (2021). Associations between physical health conditions and posttraumatic stress disorder according to age. *Aging & Mental Health*, 25(2): 234–242.

Treleaven, D.A. (2018). *Trauma-sensitive mindfulness: Practices for safe and transformative healing*. New York: WW Norton & Company.

Van den Hout, M.A. and Engelhard, I.M. (2012). How does EMDR work? *Journal of Experimental Psychopathology*, 3(5): 724–738.

Wadji, D.L., Martin-Soelch, C. and Camos, V. (2022). Can working memory account for EMDR efficacy in PTSD? *BMC Psychology*, 10: 245.

Woon, F.L. and Hedges, D.W. (2009). Amygdala volume in adults with posttraumatic stress disorder: A meta-analysis. *The Journal of Neuropsychiatry and Clinical Neurosciences*, 21(1): 5–12.

World Health Organisation (2022). *International Classification of Diseases Eleventh Revision (ICD-11)*. https://icd.who.int/browse/2024-01/mms/en#2070699808 [Accessed 12 August 2024].

Yoshii, T. (2021). The role of the thalamus in post-traumatic stress disorder. *International Journal of Molecular Sciences*, 22(4): 1730.

Zayfert, C. and Black Becker, C. (2020). *Cognitive-behavioral therapy for PTSD* (2nd ed.). New York: Guilford Press.

5

Effective support for people with complex PTSD and those diagnosed with a personality disorder

Sharon Martin-Brown

Case study

Sally's story

I've felt different all my life, as far back as I can remember. My earliest memories are not of being held or cuddled, but of being told off for 'being silly' and then being told off for crying. So, I used to hide my tears, and whenever something happened and I felt tears coming, I would escape to my bedroom so no-one could see. I felt nobody cared about me and that I had no-one who understood me.

But then I became a teenager and my body began to change, and I noticed that boys liked it. It felt like suddenly I was noticed and when I looked in the mirror at myself, I really saw the child being left behind and I was changed in ways that others were calling pretty. I have a vivid memory of being 14 and seeing one of the sixth form lads staring at my chest. Rather than shrink away with embarrassment, I pushed my chest out a bit more and licked my lips. I was startled by his response – he got all red in the face and was stammering. I remember thinking: 'I've got some power here'. It wasn't long after that, that I found myself behind the local parade of shops having sex with him. It was my first time and was over so fast. What I liked the most was him holding me. The other

DOI: 10.4324/9781003635604-5

stuff felt quite horrible to be honest, but I loved feeling his arms around me and him holding me tightly.

I felt ashamed that my first time had been like that, and I just couldn't handle that feeling. I belonged to online chat groups where girls were talking about cutting themselves and saying what a relief it was to get bad stuff out. So, I did it too. Just a little cut on the top of my arm – it hurt to begin with but gave me a feeling of relief too.

From there began a long story of boy after boy. I let them do whatever they wanted but I always made sure they held me. It made me feel as though they liked me, even if they were just getting what they wanted. Feelings of shame followed quickly each time, so the cutting became a habit to get rid of that feeling. It wasn't too long after that I fell pregnant. Those teenage boys were not careful, and neither was I. I don't even know who the dad was. I longed to have that baby, someone who would need me and who I could look after, but Mum and Dad weren't having any of it. I was marched into the doctor and then into a clinic and that was the end of that dream. I was only 15.

I hated my parents. They were telling me what to do and how to live my life, but they didn't have a clue. They argued constantly and dad would often be drunk. Mum was bitter and angry most of the time and I couldn't talk to her at all. When I was 16, Dad had been drunk every evening for about a week and I was fed up hearing them row. So, I yelled at them to shut up and Dad came storming up the stairs to me. He was yelling at me, calling me names, and something inside me broke. I just couldn't stand being in that house any longer with them and their carry-ons. A few days later, I packed a few things, stole some money out of Mum's purse and took off. I just had to get away.

I ended up on the streets. It was such a frightening and horrible time, but I did meet someone who seemed friendly and offered some help. The trouble was it really wasn't the sort of help I needed and soon turned into drug addiction and sex work. Ten long years of men taking everything and me using anything I could get my hands on to blot it out. And the cutting was my constant. It *helped when the shame became too much, which was often. I felt hopeless most of the time.*

Then one day when I ended up in the emergency department getting patched up after a particularly nasty client encounter, I met a really nice mental health nurse. She saw my self-harm scars and didn't judge me. She was kind and gave me some leaflets about rehab and treatment for emotionally unstable personality disorder. I didn't have a clue what that meant. But I think for the first time, I really thought I could change my life. That was the very start of me wanting to change, but I didn't have any idea what life could look like, so things continued as they were for a while anyway. But her words and her kindness stayed with me. I began to dream and plan. I knew it wouldn't be easy, but I so desperately wanted to get away from what I was doing and who I had become.

Eventually, I did escape. I had to move across the country to get away from those who believed they owned me as they wouldn't be happy with their money-making machine disappearing. I was housed in a hostel at first and got clean from drugs, before getting my own flat. I've written that in one sentence, but it took a long time with many ups and downs along the way. I was still cutting from time to time when things got difficult. That was so much harder to give up and in itself became a source of shame, which seems bizarre given that I first did it to get rid of shame.

Then I started having nightmares. Horrible visions that would wake me up, sweating and breathless. I also had a really bad startle reflex, anything would make me jump – a door banging, someone shouting, the roar of a motorbike. I would shake and it would take ages for me to calm down. The self-harm increased again after that as it seemed as though it was the only way to manage and to cope with the feelings I had.

One day I cut myself really badly and again needed to go to the emergency department. A mental health nurse came to talk to me and she talked about a referral into secondary services where I would be able to access treatment. She talked about Dialectical

Behaviour Therapy and at first, I thought, no I can't do therapy. I can't talk about myself and what I have done, and what I continue to do. But I did get referred and my Care Co-ordinator wanted me to do DBT. She encouraged me to think about it and put me in touch with a therapist who did another assessment. She asked me the big questions, about what I did and when and how that effected how I felt. At first, I was so embarrassed. But she didn't judge me, and I was able to relax a bit and tell her my whole story. It felt good in the end to get it all out to someone who was calm and kind.

So DBT began and I didn't like it at first. It's quite a matter-of-fact therapy, very direct and I had to record all my emotions and my self-harm on a weekly diary card. Again, up came shame about what I was doing but very quickly I was in a skills group learning new ways of managing how I felt. It was such a revelation that other things worked, instead of cutting! It wasn't too long after that, that I cut for the very last time. I'm so proud to write that statement!

When I look back on my life, I feel so sad for my early beginnings. But I have radically accepted that my life is what it is, and I cannot change my past. But I can influence my future. I continue to work hard on managing the difficult emotions that everyone feels, and I look forward to the day when I can sleep all night and no longer wake with a nightmare. I believe that day will be soon.

Introduction

This chapter builds on the knowledge gained from the previous chapter concerning post-traumatic stress disorder (PTSD) and looks specifically at the diagnosis and criteria relating to complex PTSD or C-PTSD. It will introduce the concept of how complex trauma impacts on the formation of personality and how this can manifest in adult life. Alongside discussing specific treatments available for both C-PTSD and some personality disorders, it will broaden knowledge and understanding of these complex mental health disorders.

Chapter aims

This chapter includes information and ideas relating to:

- The difference between single and complex traumas.
- The role of attachment patterns and how these are formed.
- The impact of neglect on a child.
- Understanding patient and service user's coping behaviours in times of crisis and how to give effective help.
- Helping patients and service users stabilise, to support the effectiveness of therapy.
- Specialist treatment for personality disorder and current discussions around treatment for C-PTSD.

Complex trauma

As we have discovered in Chapter 4, traumatic events impact on the brain's ability to process what has happened and how to act when a similar event either happens again or there is a likelihood that it will happen again. For example, if you are in a car accident and you are hit by a red car, your brain may become more alert and aware of other red cars on the road. This is part of keeping you safe and avoiding another accident taking place. This protective action may, however, become so generalised and severe that over the course of time, all cars may be deemed unsafe, with your brain becoming so sensitive to 'cars' in general that you decide to avoid driving altogether. This would be described as PTSD of a one trauma episode. In this chapter, we are going to look at what happens when there is more than one trauma and where repeated traumas may occur.

C-PTSD can develop in response to any of the following scenarios and events:

- Any form of childhood abuse or neglect.
- Repeated sexual abuse beginning in childhood.
- Being subjected to domestic abuse including violence, emotional and psychological abuse, financial abuse and being separated from others by means of control and coercion.
- Being involved in war, torture, sex trafficking or modern-day slavery.

The above list also indicates that in many cases, the perpetrators are known to the person, including family members and other close relationships. What is also prevalent and worthy of note is that the person is often unable to escape from the situation. This means that abuses are often recurring and potentially long-term. Alongside the PTSD symptoms of nightmares and flashbacks, the person may also develop feelings of guilt and shame, and difficulties with emotional regulation and relational issues, such as finding it hard to trust others (NHS, 2022; World Health Organisation, 2022).

The beginning of life

From the moment of birth, a baby will seek to bond or attach to its mother for survival. A baby left alone will quickly perish so babies are therefore born with the ability to obtain their caregiver's attention by crying. The aim of this is to ensure essential needs are met, such as being fed when hungry. The brain is formed with the potential for further development but there is an immediate ability for social interaction. There are some systems in the baby's brain that are fluid and adapt to the environment. One of these is the stress response.

In the first few weeks and months of life, a baby will learn how its distress signals are responded to and will learn its own systems of emotion regulation. Therefore, a mother or primary caregiver who is attentive and responds lovingly and sensitively to her baby's distress, is teaching the baby that it can experience highly emotional responses to the world and that with soothing it can be calmed again. This leads to a secure attachment with the primary caregiver (Bowlby, 2005) and from that point of having a secure base, the baby begins to learn ways to sooth and calm itself (Gerhardt, 2004).

This is not suggesting that mothers and caregivers have to give perfect care. On the contrary, as babies need months of care, the likelihood is that within that time, parents get tired and exhausted. There is also a concept of the 'good enough mother' (Winnicott, 1971). Although initially the primary caregiver may experience a sense of complete sacrifice in deference to the needs of the baby, over time the mother can allow the baby times of frustration, albeit for very short periods of time. This becomes a learning process, so the baby recognises that they are no longer part of the mother, and they begin to experience a world beyond one where the mother meets every need. Winnicott believed this was crucial to the developing brain and to the ability of the baby to see itself as an individual person, separate from the mother or primary caregiver.

A key consideration, though, is what happens when a mother is not completely attuned to the baby. This can be envisioned in terms of two ends of a scale: at one end, we can categorise the baby who has been neglected and at the other end, is the baby with overly intrusive parents. The neglected baby may have a depressed mother who finds it hard to attune to and read her baby's distress signals. The baby may therefore receive only limited interaction – only being picked up to be fed and changed, and this taking place with little demonstration of warmth or care in the mother's touch. The baby will learn there is no point protesting too much as it gains no response, so cries less. In turn, the mother may find the child easier to deal with as it does not cry so often.

At the other end of the scale could be a depressed parent who struggles to attune to her baby, but this parent may have a rougher and less sensitive approach to the baby. One day she may be heightened in her own emotional arousal, being loud and overly expressive to the baby, and on other days, she may experience flatness and detachment in mood. The baby will be confused and will be unable to predict what sort of responses to expect to its distress signals. The baby may also stay in an overly aroused state itself, without the ability to soothe and calm itself (Gerhardt, 2004). These latter states can then translate into an insecure attachment system, being anxious or avoidant, with each having an impact on the formulation of the personality into adult life.

These early-life experiences lay down the foundations of how the adult person will relate in the world and if early-life development has a poor trajectory into anxious or avoidant attachment systems, then that person may be at risk of developing C-PTSD or a personality disorder. In summary, a child needs safety and consistency to be able to develop the skills needed in regulation of the self, as well as to live and to live well, in the external world (Porges, 2011).

The developed adult

A person who has been subjected to the trauma of neglect may present with any number of the following signs and symptoms in adulthood:

- Persistent difficulties with relationships.
- Substance and alcohol misuse (as numbing agents).
- Self-harm and suicidal thoughts and actions.

- Highly emotional outbursts at minor stressors.
- Depressive symptoms – low, flat mood, low motivation, lack of self-care leading to self-neglect, over- or under-eating.
- Rumination about specific events.

The person may also describe experiencing:

- Flashbacks and nightmares with strong emotional qualities.
- Hypervigilance and being constantly on guard.
- Symptoms relating to dissociating – losing track of time, feeling disconnected from others, having a sense of unreality in the present moment.
- Not being able to experience joy or pleasure in everyday activities.
- Feelings of worthlessness, guilt, shame, defeat, anger and sadness.
- Intense pain without an identifiable organic cause.

These lists are not exhaustive but form part of the International Classification of Diseases (ICD-11) criteria for diagnosing C-PTSD (World Health Organisation, 2022).

Looking at a similar case where the diagnosis is of personality disorder, this can include similar signs and symptoms as seen in the DSM-5 (American Psychiatric Association, 2013). The person would need to evidence five of these symptoms before a diagnosis is given:

1. Frantic efforts to avoid abandonment.
2. Unstable and intense relationships.
3. Identity disturbance.
4. Impulsivity in at least two areas (sex, substance misuse, reckless driving, spending and binge eating).
5. Recurrent suicidal or self-harming actions.
6. Affective instability.
7. Chronic feelings of emptiness.
8. Inappropriate intense anger or difficulty controlling anger.
9. Transient stress-related paranoid ideation or severe dissociation symptoms.

The signs and symptoms of C-PTSD and the specific criteria named for diagnosis in borderline personality disorder (BPD) overlap and are very similar. BPD is sometimes known as emotionally unstable personality disorder (EUPD) with a key aspect of this diagnosis being the identification of generalised emotional sensitivity and emotional dysregulation. Great care needs to be exercised before a diagnosis is made, and this needs to be done specifically by a psychiatrist or psychologist. It is also worth noting that the need to work with the individual to establish stability is similar whether the person is diagnosed as having a personality disorder or C-PTSD.

Kulkarni (2017) identified that trauma plays a key role in the development of both C-PTSD and BPD. Given a current lack of differentiation between these conditions, and the high stigma faced by people with BPD, it is suggested that using the diagnostic term 'complex post-traumatic stress disorder' is preferable as it decreases stigma and provides a trauma-informed approach for patients. Nonetheless, ongoing concerns about the impact of a personality disorder diagnosis exist. Nicki (2016) argues that the common use of the psychiatric diagnosis of BPD with female survivors of chronic childhood trauma poses a serious risk of pathologising their life experiences, along with their subsequent coping behaviours and survival strategies. It is suggested that it is highly likely that diagnostic and clinical practices related to BPD are significantly informed by cultural and gender norms. Therefore, we could argue that health practitioners and society as a whole need to be open to an empathic understanding of the life experiences, social situations and loss of developmentally enriching opportunities in their childhoods, of survivors of longer-term abuse and neglect.

Meanwhile, Walker and Kulkarni (2020) have developed this discussion by noting how debilitating and stigmatising a diagnosis of BPD is for many people. They argue that viewing BPD as a personality disorder involves conceptualising it as a group of symptoms, rather than as a way of responding to trauma, whereas such attitudes are less common in disorders that are identified as trauma-based, such as C-PTSD. Walker and Kulkarni therefore argue that 're-framing BPD as a trauma-spectrum disorder could improve clinician attitudes, help reduce stigma and inform trauma-conscious treatment strategies' (Walker and Kulkarni, 2020: 238), ultimately contributing to improved outcomes for these patients.

Understanding the patient in crisis

There are some patients and service users who appear to go from crisis to crisis on a constant basis. Linehan (1993) names this as 'unrelenting crises'. It can be exhausting for health and care practitioners to try and support the person during these times, because it often feels as though one thing after another happens, and that the need for support is persistent and unremitting. We therefore need to try to understand what is happening to the person at these times.

If the person you are supporting has been diagnosed with either C-PTSD or a personality disorder, it is likely that they are highly sensitive to their emotions. They can also be sensitive to words and gestures when interacting with others; when those interactions appear negative or critical, the patient's emotional responses will be higher, matching the intensity of their feelings. As a result, minor criticisms and negative interactions have every potential for escalation.

The following example from Sally's history helps to illustrate this.

One Saturday night I attended the emergency department after I was beaten up. A nurse came in to do clinical observations and I had to roll up my sleeve for my blood pressure to be taken. She saw my self-harm scars and tutted. Not a word was said, but that 'tut' said everything. I was so embarrassed and ashamed of myself. I wanted life to end right in that moment. I don't know how I stayed and got patched up, I wanted to crawl into a hole and die.

In this example, we can see the devastation to Sally of being tutted at and how her response to this was to want her life to end. There is such a marked level of reactivity due to the sensitivity that Sally experiences.

Think again about the impact of past experiences. The person in front of you as an adult, may have grown up in a home environment where their emotions were not taken seriously, or where they were joked about, laughed at and even punished or ignored. This is an emotionally invalidating environment. We have emotional reactions to stimuli every day. Sometimes these are pleasant, such as feeling calm at seeing the sunrise, or experiencing joy when listening to music. Sometimes though, our emotions might be evaluated as being negative or bad, for example, when we react with feelings of sadness or anger. Imagine being told to *'cheer up'* if you feel sad about a recent loss, or perhaps being told to *'grow up: only babies cry'*. If children are regularly and constantly told 'don't feel that', or they have the message that their emotions are wrong or too much, they can grow up not trusting how they feel.

Emotions come from a primal part of our brain (Siegel and Solomon, 2003). In evolutionary terms, we had emotions before we could talk, and all emotions play a part in keeping us safe and helping us to maintain our place within our community or family group. Emotions consist of an inner experience (what we feel), which leads to an outer, noticeable expression, giving rise to urges for action. So, if we are told by our primary caregivers not to feel as we do, or not to trust how we feel, we learn to deny an intrinsic part of ourselves which is needed for survival. However, denying or suppressing emotions does not make them disappear. Instead, they can become stronger, and the brain learns that the emotions need to be 'bigger' for us to take notice of them and to take the action needed to protect us. Ultimately, a patient or service user may become highly sensitive to their emotions, as well as experiencing a higher intensity of emotions on a regular basis.

Understanding this sensitivity and intensity helps in beginning to understand how small things can quickly escalate for some patients and service users. It has become part of a natural, protective response due to forming sensitivity in early life. The following sections explore a range of tools and approaches, which may help people to regulate and manage their emotions.

Tools for now: small changes that can make a big difference

As a health and care practitioner, you may already have your own toolkit of skills that you bring to your role, but it is helpful to go back to basics and understand why such tools are important when working with people with C-PTSD and those with emotional dysregulation.

Listening skills

Each patient or service user needs to know that you understand how they feel. You can show understanding by listening, which gives the person time to tell you what is happening to them and how it makes them feel. Remember the patient in front of you may have had many years of being told *'don't feel that'* and yet they are in front of you, taking a risk in sharing their inner world. They are trusting you not to join the group of people who have invalidated their emotions throughout their lives. Avoid asking too many questions and allow space for the person to formulate what they want to tell you. When appropriate, you could ask an open question to allow them to further expand or reflect on what they have said. Using paraphrasing or summarising shows that you have listened and are checking your understanding.

Non-verbal communication

Think about what your body is communicating. The acronym SOLER may help here (Egan, 2001):

1. Sit squarely
2. Open posture
3. Lean in slightly
4. Eye contact
5. Relax

Each of these five aspects of non-verbal communication helps to ensure that our focus is fully orientated on the person in front of us, thus demonstrating that we value them and their story.

Validation

Your ability to validate the person's emotional experience could be the first reparative step in their recovery. Remember that they may have had many years of having their feelings belittled or being told their emotions are wrong, so think about being able to use validation and affirmation as part of routine conversations, such as: 'Yes, you will feel sadness at that loss', or 'Yes, you would feel angry if that person was rude to you'. Being validated may be a completely new experience for them, and can be highly reparative with potential for strengthening the therapeutic relationship between you.

Boundaries

Establish boundaries within each appointment, including the reason for meeting and how long the appointment is. Misattunement over boundaries can lead to frustration and can be easily avoided. If you are providing a short check in call or appointment, this needs to be said at the outset. Don't let a patient get well along in what could potentially be a long story if you don't have time to listen to the end. It doesn't have to be negative to say, 'I have 15 minutes today', if you can add: 'but I can see you need to talk, so why don't we book in a longer appointment for next week?' The ability to work in this way will vary according to setting, although it is always important that we are clear about what we can offer and whether there are limits on our available time and relevant expertise.

Helping the person prepare for therapy

Sometimes there are misconceptions about what is going to happen when a patient starts therapy. It is useful to understand what type of therapy the person is having, and why. You don't need an in-depth knowledge of the therapy, but it can help to understand whether it is a skills-based approach, a relational approach or an analytical approach.

Many therapies need the person to be able to reflect on or to manage complex and difficult emotions as they arise. The exception to this would be dialectical behaviour therapy (DBT) (Linehan, 1993), which has been specifically designed for the complex patient who does not have those skills. DBT is explored in more detail later in this chapter.

Patients do need enough stability to be able to withstand therapy. It may be a strange and contentious thought, but therapy is often de-stabilising. In trauma treatment especially, the focus is looking at past, painful episodes of the person's life, along with the emotions surrounding events, the negative thoughts that have developed and grown around the events and any coping mechanisms and patterns of behaviour, which may have been reinforced over time. This can be a painful time as the person re-encounters events. Maintaining stability is essential to withstanding what happens in therapy and for recovery from trauma to be possible. As a health and care practitioner, you can do much to help keep this stability as your patient progresses in treatment. Here are some ideas to consider:

1. Keep regular appointments with your patient. Don't assume that as your patient is in therapy, they no longer need you. They do. A boundaried relationship with you may be a safe space as they make sense of new insights, skills and ways of being in the world.
2. Make sure the person has a crisis and safety plan documented and prepared in advance, in case of need. If you are prepared for instability and know what to do if this occurs, the destructive elements of any crisis are more likely to be limited.
3. Think about guiding the person in preparing a soothing-kit or 'health first aid kit' before therapy starts. Things for the kit can be based on sensory experience and can include:
   a. Books and music to listen to
   b. Pictures to look at
   c. Essential oils to smell

    d. Sugary, sharp or sour food to taste

    e. Soft material to touch

4. Consider that there may be reinforcements happening in the patient's environment that maintain less effective coping behaviours. Involving family members in psycho-education about the therapy may therefore be helpful.

Specialist treatments: longer-term approaches

There are a variety of treatment options for personality disorder, so at assessment, we need to understand where the person's difficulties are most prevalent and offer treatment and talking therapies with those difficulties in mind. Guidance from NICE (2009) states that for women who are suicidal and who self-harm, DBT is recommended.

DBT is a structured approach that encompasses one-to-one therapy, a weekly skills group, telephone skills coaching between sessions and therapists attending a weekly consultation meeting. Programmes are usually for 1 year and the patient is required to access all domains of the therapy and be willing to work on goals that make life worth living as well as being committed to reduce and stop all self-harming and suicidal behaviours. Willingness to practise skills and complete homework outside of one-to-one and skills group therapy sessions is also a pre-requisite. There are four domains of DBT within which the skills focus is on Mindfulness, Emotion Regulation, Distress Tolerance and Interpersonal Effectiveness. In essence, the skills deficit described in Linehan's (1993) biosocial model is addressed within these four domains as the person learns the skills not taught or absorbed earlier in life. This therapy can have a stabilising effect on the patient as they become more skilful at coping with life events, with the aim of achieving personal goals that make life worth living for them.

Often DBT is used as a pre-cursor before other trauma therapy is attempted. However, there is currently a growing evidence base for treating trauma within DBT using a prolonged exposure protocol (Harned, 2022). Harned worked within the model of DBT under Linehan for many years and found that there was a category of client who were too high risk for trauma work to be attempted as a first-line intervention. Yet it was the complexity of the trauma they had experienced, which caused them to be engaging in high-risk behaviours. In response to this 'Catch-22' situation, Harned developed a structured method and model that incorporates all the tenets of DBT with trauma-focused treatment being attempted once a level of stability has been attained.

Summary of learning points

This chapter has explored the following theoretical and practical approaches to understanding and supporting people living with C-PTSD and those diagnosed with emotionally unstable (and similar) personality disorders:

- The origin of symptoms of personality disorders lies in childhood trauma over which the individual had no control.
- Control can, however, be regained by the adult survivor of childhood trauma by enabling the processing of emotions and improved emotional regulation in adulthood, which generally leads to a more satisfying life with fewer crises.
- Being listened to, feeling heard and being validated are essential for wellbeing for people experiencing the symptoms of C-PTSD and those diagnosed with personality disorders with emotional dysregulation.
- The trauma that these people have experienced has altered the way they interact with others and the world. This is not the person's fault but relates to the way their brains processed the trauma.
- DBT has been identified as an effective therapy for some people who are living with the long-term effects of complex trauma.

Questions for reflection and discussion

1. Patients and service users have described experiencing discrimination against people with a diagnosis of personality disorder or emotional dysregulation. Identify how any such discrimination towards patients and service users accessing your organisation's services could be challenged and reduced.

2. There are similarities in symptoms experienced by people with EUPD, C-PTSD and BPD. Identify the elements of an effective and helpful response to a person presenting with any diagnosis involving emotional dysregulation?

3. How can you adapt your approach within a short appointment to enable a person to know that they have been heard and that their feelings are validated?

4. Some patients and service users use self-harm as a strategy for coping with strong emotions. How might you adopt a non-judgemental approach to advising patients about the potential physical risks of self-harm (for example, sepsis) as well as about trying some alternative ways of managing emotions?

5. What sort of training would you and your colleagues need to broaden your understanding of these diagnoses? How could this translate into an improved service for your patients?

Recommended follow-up reading

Balmer, A., Sambrook, L., Roks, H., Ashley-Mudie, P., Tait, J., Bu, C., McIntyre, J.C., Shetty, A., Nathan, R. and Saini, P. (2024). Perspectives of service users and carers with lived experience of a diagnosis of personality disorder: A qualitative study. *Journal of Psychiatric and Mental Health Nursing*, 31(1): 55–65.

Danquah, A.N. and Berry, K. (2013). *Attachment theory in adult mental health: A guide to clinical practice*. Abingdon: Routledge.

Javed, A. and Sharma, R. (2023). "It's all in the head" well! not always: Mental health patients are not immune to physical pain. *British Journal of Psychiatry Open*, 9(S1): S123–S123.

Mattocks, N. (2025). Lived experience perspective on internalised stigma and the EUPD diagnosis. *Journal of Psychiatric and Mental Health Nursing*, 32(1): 248–251.

References

American Psychiatric Association, DSM-5 Task Force. (2013). *Diagnostic and statistical manual of mental disorders: DSM-5™* (5th ed.). Washington, DC: American Psychiatric Association Publishing.

Bowlby, J. (2005). *A secure base*. Abingdon: Routledge Classics.

Egan, G. (2001). *The skilled helper* (7th ed. s.l.). Belmont: Wadsworth Publishing Co Inc.

Gerhardt, S. (2004). *Why love matters*. East Hove: Routledge.

Harned, M. (2022). *Treating trauma in dialectical behaviour therapy*. New York: The Guildford Press.

Kulkarni, J. (2017). Complex PTSD – A better description for borderline personality disorder? *Australasian Psychiatry*, 25(4): 333–335.

Linehan, M.M. (1993). *Cognitive behavioural treatment of borderline personality disorder*. New York: The Guildford Press.

NHS (2022). *Complex PTSD – Post traumatic stress disorder*. https://www.nhs.uk/mental-health/conditions/post-traumatic-stress-disorder-ptsd/complex/ [Accessed 28th January 2025].

NICE (2009). *Clinical Guideline (CG78). Borderline personality disorder: Recognition and management*. https://www.nice.org.uk/guidance/cg78/chapter/Recommendations#assessment-and-management-by-community-mental-health-services [Accessed 28th January 2025].

Nicki, A. (2016). Borderline personality disorder, discrimination, and survivors of chronic childhood trauma. *IJFAB: International Journal of Feminist Approaches to Bioethics*, 9(1): 218–245.

Porges, S.W. (2011). *The polyvagal theory: Neurophysiological foundations of emotions, attachment, communication and self-regulation*. New York/London: W.W. Norton and Co.

Siegel, D.J. and Solomon, M. (2003). *Healing trauma: Attachment, mind, body and brain*. London: W.W. Norton & Company.

Walker, P. and Kulkarni, J. (2020). Re-framing borderline personality disorder. *Australasian Psychiatry*, 28(2): 237–238.

Winnicott, D.W. (1971). *Playing and reality*. New York: Basic Books.

World Health Organisation (2022). *International classification of diseases for mortality and morbidity*. https://icd.who.int/browse/2024-01/mms/en#585833559 [Accessed 30th January 2025].

6 | Supporting traumatised individuals

Covering the B.A.C.E.S

Tamsin Black and Sarah Housden

Case study

Samaira's story

When I was in Primary School, a friend of my father came from Bangladesh to live in our spare bedroom. This meant that there was always an adult at home for us, even when our parents were out working. We got to hear lots of stories of our father from when he was growing up and Uncle was fun and often helpful. A few years later, when I was 9 years old, my older sister left home for university, and I finally got to move into her little room and stopped sharing with my little sisters.

My Uncle soon offered to help me with my homework in my room, as he had done with my older sister. My parents were very grateful and studying seriously made me feel very grown up. I felt special at first, but then he began making comments about my body and how I walked and talked. My parents and siblings found this funny but his attitude to me made me feel embarrassed and confused. Then, he began coming into my room after every one else was asleep in their beds. He did lots of sexual things to me and got me to do lots of disgusting and sometimes painful things that I didn't understand at the time, but I knew they were wrong and that I didn't want to do them. Uncle often threatened we

DOI: 10.4324/9781003635604-6

would soon 'go all the way'. He told me that if I said anything, my parents would get in trouble, my father would surely have a heart attack, and my sister would have to leave university. The more time passed, the harder it was for me to tell anyone. A short time after my eleventh birthday, I got my period. I got really scared that he would now think me old enough to rape, but when he found out about my period, he stopped visiting me at night. It took me a while to realise that he wasn't going to do it again.

I felt very confused for a long time, Uncle stayed living with us and would sometimes try to kiss me, intimidate me and say things in front of other people which upset me. He could make me feel scared or ashamed, just by looking at me. Then, I started to worry that he had shifted his attention to my younger sisters. I looked for signs of this and skipped last lessons to avoid leaving them alone with him. I tried to stay awake at night. My family used to get cross with me and say I had no friends. I couldn't join in with my friends' gossip about teachers, their after-school clubs and make up, or explain why.

Then, I started skipping school, just because it was all too much. When my Form teacher called a meeting with my parents, I told them what had been happening and my fears for my little sisters. My parents didn't believe me and said I was 'an ungrateful girl' and was blaming Uncle to get myself out of trouble. I thought my school would call the Police and have Uncle taken away, and that would convince my parents. School called Social Services, and I remember the anger in mum's eyes and her silence as we waited. They said we could go home if my mother and father promised that Uncle would stay away until he was interviewed. Once home, I was sent to my room, and I wanted to die.

When the Social Worker came to our house, I was so ashamed and fearful of saying the wrong thing, I couldn't speak to them. Later, my younger sisters and brothers told me the Social Worker had talked to each of them and left. I didn't hear anything more about it and after the weekend, I went back to school. My mother told me that Uncle had been so offended at the threat to his reputation and liberty that he wanted nothing to do with us anymore. My *father seemed sad and my mother disapproving of me. Everything changed. I felt that my parents would never forgive me, especially as things got tougher without his money and practical help.*

I found out from my teacher that Social Services decided to drop any investigation due to my parents' evident fear and shame, as well as the news that Uncle was no longer living with us. They were fearful of causing inter-racial offence. They could see I was a bright girl, doing well at school and said I could have counselling if I wanted to. I didn't want to, I felt too guilty and just got stuck back into school and trying to do well.

I'm home for the Easter holidays from university. I'm so tired, I don't belong anywhere. The only thing I like there is my course, no one has contacted me, and I've got nothing to post online to get a response from my friends there. Everyone at home is just polite, nothing to say, and it's awkward. I've been scratching and cutting my thighs every now and then since Uncle left and it seemed that everyone started hating me. Not so much at Uni, but this is the first time I've cut my wrists. I was feeling so lonely and helpless, but also angry and frustrated. I don't want this to be my life. I'm so tired – it is a long time since I slept well at night. Now that I am at the Emergency Department, I feel so stupid. I don't want to die, not just because it's forbidden in my religion. I want to live a good life. I just cannot see a way forward.

Introduction

Samaira is a victim of childhood sexual abuse. In common with many childhood abuse survivors, her developmental path has been distorted by acts of emotional and sexual abuse, endured over a prolonged period of confusing feelings, difficult to understand responses and behaviours, and disturbed relationships. Emotional, physical and sexual abuse in childhood commonly involves coercive control (Stark and Hester, 2019) and emotional and relational manipulation. There are many idiosyncratic factors that contribute to the victim's risk of social isolation, unhelpful views of themselves, other people and their own future, which guide their behaviour and developmental opportunities. In this chapter, we will return to Samaira to help us understand which elements of her story may have worked to increase or decrease her vulnerability to complex post-traumatic stress disorder (PTSD) (Rosenfield et al., 2018; WHO, 2019), and what health and social care staff might have done to help her.

Chapter aims

This chapter seeks to promote understanding of factors that increase and decrease vulnerability in people who have experienced trauma. We have selected easy-to-access resources to support meaningful interventions at every healthcare and social services encounter for the wellbeing of service users and staff. The chapter includes information and ideas relating to:

- Responding to a disclosure of abuse.
- Trauma-stabilising techniques compatible with single or short-term contacts with traumatised individuals.
- Values Led Behavioural Activation principles, presented as *a newly adapted B.A.C.E.S. framework* to guide assessment and intervention in a way that better supports resilience within the service user and their network.

Contemporary theory and practice

Throughout this chapter, it will be helpful to keep at the forefront of your mind, the principles of trauma-informed care (TIC), namely safety, trust, choice, collaboration, empowerment and cultural considerations (Office for Health Improvement and Disparities, 2022). This chapter will consider approaches that non-psychotherapy and non-trauma specialist practitioners could use to help someone like Samaira to mobilise factors that decrease her vulnerability and that support her continuing recovery from earlier trauma.

Other chapters in this book discuss therapeutic interventions that directly target the processing of traumatic events to relieve intrusive experiences such as flashbacks and hypervigilance, and to manage and reduce distressing arousal[1]. Such approaches help the traumatised person to make sense of and overcome, life-restricting behavioural patterns such as avoidance. Small steps which the service user can take, are especially important to recovery as there are many barriers to effective psychotherapeutic treatment, not least those due to long waiting lists and varying treatment availability across the United Kingdom. Furthermore, aspects of treatment may turn out to be intolerable to some individuals, even when other barriers are overcome. For example, exposure to reminders of the trauma and to intense emotions, as part of reprocessing methods, are not always acceptable to people who are struggling to regulate everyday emotions[2], or to people who have difficulties with trust and those who experience deep shame (Lewis et al., 2020).

Despite agreement that trauma-focussed psychotherapy is the frontline treatment for trauma-associated presentations of distress, it has been estimated that between one-third and one half of PTSD patients do not optimally respond to these treatments and continue to display persistent PTSD symptoms (Keyan et al., 2024). This is what drives the following chapter content and our encouragement for health and social care staff to think of every contact as an opportunity to provide interpersonal experiences and to reinforce strategies that support the inherent resilience and available resources of the traumatised person.

Childhood sexual abuse in a person's history should not exclude them from accessing more readily available approaches, though often it does. Health and social care professionals may feel inhibited by the awful reality of the traumatised person's story, and so be reluctant to offer the same care they offer to others or be worried about making matters worse or about starting something which they cannot follow through (Sweeney et al., 2018).

The strategies we will describe here might help someone with difficulties occurring because of earlier traumatic experiences, especially those relating to sleep, mood, loneliness or unhelpful behavioural strategies, such as avoidance. They are in keeping with TIC and other new ways of conceptualising human distress like The Power Threat Meaning Framework, helping us to understand and stay on side with the person in front of us (Johnstone et al., 2018).

Survivors of sexual assault with comorbid depression appear to have poorer outcomes even following specialist trauma treatment than individuals with PTSD alone (Resick, 2001). In addition, trauma-related guilt has been found to be more strongly associated with depression than PTSD in treatment-seeking rape victims (Bennice et al., 2001). A trauma-informed approach to coping day to day is needed, in which we ask the person in front of us *'how can we help you with what you are dealing with?'* rather than *'how can we fix you?'* This chapter and accompanying resources seek to empower you to develop your thinking and practice, to be and to feel more effective, in every encounter with a traumatised person.

Survivors of complex trauma often experience feelings of hopelessness and a lack of belief that anything within their control might improve their situation. There may be issues with tolerating negative or strongly positive emotions; with attentional flexibility, relationships or achieving a state of bodily calm. Indeed, people living in the wake of complex trauma are at risk of having their traumatic experiences unrecognised and being mis-diagnosed with psychiatric disorders such as emotionally unstable personality disorder (EUPD) or borderline personality disorder (BPD), bipolar affective disorder, chronic depression or dysthymia (Rosenfield et al., 2018; WHO, 2019).

It is often the case that people presenting with self-regulation challenges alongside difficulties in interpersonal relations, have had a traumatic past (Dale et al., 2017). Zanarini et al. (1989) reported that 84% of people diagnosed with BPD retrospectively described experiences of bi-parental neglect and emotional abuse before aged 18. The effect of living with such difficulties can be catastrophic: compared to the general population. For a range of reasons, people labelled as having a personality disorder have their lives cut shorter, with men dying 17.7 years prematurely and women's lives being an average of 18.7 years shorter (Fok et al., 2012). Personality disorder programmes are intensive and are usually offered over a period of at least 1 year. Thankfully, there is now a far greater emphasis on a history of trauma as part of the developmental course of personality disorders, including those occurring alongside, or because of unrecognised neurodiversity. There is greater emphasis on what we need to be doing to adjust our own behaviour and the environments in which we deliver care, to better accommodate the needs and sensitivities of others.

Although there is now widespread recognition that TIC is vital, it is not always clear how best to resource staff, so that they feel confident to enter into conversations with trauma survivors. Healthcare practitioners are often orientated towards tasks and throughput (Sharp et al., 2018) rather than the emotional experience and learning of being with another person in their distress. An emotionally containing and yet pragmatic approach is needed. Lamb et al. (2018) have emphasised the importance of routinely training health and social care staff to work in a trauma-informed way.

In the United Kingdom, the Department for Levelling Up, Housing and Communities (2023) concluded that the evidence-based principles of TIC needed widespread implementation. The TIC approach recognises self-harm as a maladaptive coping mechanism (Brereton and McGlinchey, 2019). Bulford et al. (2024) highlighted the challenges of working in a trauma-informed way, with people who have experienced trauma. In their analysis, they reviewed feedback from primary care staff who described feeling frustrated, doubtful of their abilities and overwhelmed by their work. Clear guidelines for managing disclosure of abuse are available and presented here with further literature and resources to develop practitioner confidence.

Responding to disclosure

Some people may choose not to disclose, and it is important to highlight that people do not have to answer screening questions if they do not want to. Often, we are working without really knowing what may have happened to a person to account for their presentation. TIC encourages us to apply these principles to everyone, in the knowledge that full disclosure may be too difficult or inappropriate especially in briefer health and social care encounters. However, if someone does share experiences of trauma or abuse, Sweeney et al. (2018) suggests it can be helpful to respond in the following ways:

- Provide reassurance and encouragement that disclosure is helpful and a positive thing.
- Do not ask for specific details about the trauma they may have experienced.
- Ask about their experiences of telling people in the past, and whether people have been helpful?
- Offer support around trauma and complete a referral to trauma services if required.
- Check that the person is currently safe.
- And check their emotional state on conclusion of the encounter.

Herman's tri-phasic model

A widely practised model for post-traumatic psychotherapeutic intervention is Herman's tri-phasic model (Herman, 2022). In this section, we will draw on the first phase of this highly researched and validated protocol. It is consistent and easily accessible to the non-specialist and will support your practice of TIC at every encounter. Recourse to impactful self-soothing techniques has been shown to increase the compassion and reduce the strain of the workforce and trauma survivors alike (Hunsaker et al., 2015; Kelly and Todd, 2017; Rushforth et al., 2023; Saunders et al., 2023).

Herman's tri-phasic model provides a structured approach to helping individuals heal from complex trauma, including survivors of sexual violence and is predicated on the idea that this will be achieved in the context of a strong therapeutic relationship based on trust and safety. Within TIC, we understand that the actions of traumatised individuals (including self-harm) may be understood as efforts to avoid, block out or erase traumatic memories.

The three phases of Herman's model are outlined below. The techniques of Phase One aim to establish sufficient safety to allow more helpful experiences and coping resources to develop. These are a pre-requisite for the processing of traumatic experiences into a more coherent and self-supporting narrative of past events. In this way, the individual can gain a sense of mastery and control over their history and their lives here and now. Intrusive memories and high levels of arousal are reduced as is the need for avoidant strategies that ultimately sustain fear and life-limiting beliefs and assumptions.

Safety and stabilisation

This initial phase focuses on creating a secure and stable environment, even if just in the present moment for the individual, both physically and emotionally. It involves establishing trust and supporting them to develop coping mechanisms to manage symptoms and regulate their emotions. This phase is helpful for health and social care staff, including first responders, and could helpfully be implemented within non-psychotherapy specialist encounters with traumatised individuals.

Remembrance and mourning

In this phase, the focus shifts to remembering and processing the traumatic memories. This involves exploring the trauma, acknowledging the associated losses (for example, loss of safety, trust or sense of self) and experiencing and expressing related emotions (such as anger, sadness, and guilt) in the safe and supportive environment of regular psychotherapeutic sessions.

Although details of past events are unlikely to be entered into in everyday encounters, understanding these themes without probing may help the traumatised individual's preoccupations, when presenting in crisis, to be more understandable to themselves and others.

Reconnection

The final phase involves reconnecting with others, including meaningful activities and a range of aspects of life. This stage focuses on rebuilding a sense of self, developing a more positive identity and integrating the experiences of the trauma into a coherent narrative of self. Arguably, we see these efforts and successes in the stories of traumatised individuals who we encounter, as they continually seek to strive and re-engage, to cope with and improve their lives, often in the wake of continuing and variably intense distress.

As is the case with recovery from traumatic events, the three phases of specialist treatment are not necessarily linear. Individuals may move backwards and forwards between them. We believe that this work takes place not only in structured psychological therapy encounters; it is not something done to a traumatised person but rather, is a process that is either encouraged or discouraged in day-to-day life. TIC practice is consistent with Phase One, and this can be enhanced through training in ideas and techniques for a diverse range of professionals. Baranowsky and Gentry (2015) have helpfully described a range of approaches and techniques to support Phase One work in everyday encounters with traumatised people, including those impacted by intrusive reminders of the trauma, heightened arousal and avoidant coping strategies.

As Samaira told her story, the Triage nurse noticed her shallow breathing and tearfulness. Samaira said that she kept coming over hot and dizzy. The Triage Nurse had available a summary sheet of some grounding exercises (see Chapter 4 and the Trauma Research UK reference in the Follow-up Reading section in this chapter) and demonstrated how they could be practised there and then. It took less than 10 minutes to do this, and Samaira quietly practised one of them while she waited to be seen. Such grounding techniques are understood to help a person to regain control and achieve calm and are thought to do so by interrupting anxious and otherwise unhelpful thinking processes. Phase One strategies like this have the potential to provide immediate benefit if they resonate with the trauma sufferer and are shared by a compassionate person.

Ideas from values led behavioural activation (BA)

Contemporary applications of a learning theory-informed approach called behavioural activation (BA) have shown effectiveness as a treatment, as an individual therapy, group therapy and manualised self-help, originally for low mood but also for people with symptoms of post-traumatic stress (Etherton and Farley, 2022; Jakupcak, 2020). BA has been delivered as a 4-6-10-12 week, weekly intervention. Read et al. (2016) described a single session format delivered to carers with promising outcomes. As BA practice is helpfully tied to individual values, faith-adapted versions have been developed in partnership with the Latino Community in the United States (Kanter et al., 2015) and successfully adapted to incorporate Islamic teaching with and for Muslims in the United Kingdom (Mir et al., 2015, 2019, 2023).

We are not proposing here that manualised BA is applicable to every health and social care setting, although it may be suitable for some contexts and training is available. BA is presented here in terms of the phrase and mnemonic of 'Back to B.A.C.E.S.' representing Body, Achievement, Connection, Enjoyment and Spirituality. When we say 'Back to', we seek to ground the health and social care practitioner in easily accessible skills consistent with those acquired through their training and practice and our common humanity, thus enabling all of us to engage more purposefully with and support the resilience and adaptive coping of the traumatised individual in our care.

BA is predicated on the learning theory principle that the key to changing how we feel is help that supports us to change what we do. As we go through life, we acquire behavioural patterns that help us cope with emotional distress in the short term but keep us stuck over time, such as avoidance, or self-criticism. The key to working out what might be helpful lies in what precedes and follows the behaviour (or emotional state) we want to change. By getting in touch with our values (what matters here and now, hopes, intentions, the big picture) and striving to act in line with them, we can find strength to act (behave), in line with them, and not our mood or distress. One reason why we are sharing these ideas here was that help seeking often happens in the wake of a crisis of coping. Crises are moments of disruption and could afford opportunities for what researchers call 'post-traumatic growth' (Domhardt et al., 2015; Reksoprodjo, 2023). Anxious individuals avoid change, disruption and uncertainty. Moments of crisis may be risky but may also carry opportunity to rethink, reorientate or less helpfully, to be confirmed in a negative and life-limiting perspective. The aftermath of a crisis may bring relief in some way, but this is often unpredictable and demanding of change. We offer these ideas, in the hope that the reader will find the relevance to their context and adapt them to their own practice.

It would be ill-advised if you cannot give time, to encourage a person to talk about their experiences of trauma and its effects. They may be unwilling or unable to talk about past events or once started might find the material difficult to contain. If unhelpful beliefs and guiding assumptions the person carries about what happened to them, remain unchecked or are even confirmed, health and social care encounters may be unwittingly counterproductive (Ozer et al., 2003).

Samaira was forced by her circumstances and the age at which the abuse occurred to purposefully manage her situation alone, until she became concerned for the wellbeing of her younger sisters. Only then did she seek help, and help did not materialise. We see her then striving again to cope alone and with some success. The learning over this time shaped her subsequent coping strategies. We see a combination of poor self-care, high responsibility taking, avoidance, social withdrawal and self-criticism leading to isolation and overwhelm.

BA encourages people to think about their wellbeing when planning meaningful activities. Rather than waiting to feel like doing something, individuals are encouraged to see patterns of avoidance and inactivity as understandable, albeit unhelpful symptoms of their distress, which can be counteracted by doing more of what matters to them. Over-learned or seemingly hard-wired ways of responding to emotional experience and other stimuli in the moment can be recognised and resisted and more adaptive strategies modelled or called to action.

Benefits of implementing BA in complex trauma

Therefore, an orientation to BA, even or perhaps especially in moments of crisis, may play a valuable part in recalling factors that decrease vulnerability to complex trauma responses (resilience, resources and relationships) and increase resilience through social, physical and relational dimensions of healthy functioning. It helps the individual to establish healthier daily rhythms that regulate mood and emotion and works against learned helplessness and social isolation.

Challenges of implementing BA in complex trauma

A trauma-sensitive approach is needed. Standard BA techniques may not account for dissociation, hypervigilance or emotional flashbacks, which are often present in complex trauma. It is still worth trying this approach though, as being believed and invested in are strong motivators for people with complex trauma who may not be used to this type of motivation. Small gains in terms of positive reinforcement and feelings of agency and control, as well as routine and purpose, can lead to better sleep alongside improved relationships and greater investment in the future.

Emotional readiness is important when it comes to reengaging with activity and some individuals may struggle with motivation or feel overwhelmed. Modifications and flexibility in the implementation of activities, as well as in the delivery of the elements of the BA programme, together with therapeutic support, are key to helping traumatised individuals to begin therapy and to move forward at a comfortable pace.

People impacted by developmental experiences of trauma require interventions that process traumatic memories, allowing them to be coherently stored by the brain as having occurred in the past. However, when presented with a person in distress who states clearly that they do not want to or feel able to talk about traumatic events, engaging with the impact of the trauma on their day-to-day experience can be very helpful. People are rarely completely passive but are generally engaged in active coping day to day. It can be helpful to understand the whole person and recognising knowledge and skills from other areas of living and learning, which can make a real difference, as BA can be highly beneficial for individuals with complex trauma if adapted to their needs. It provides a structure that counteracts avoidance and dwelling on the past. It helps to restore a sense of normalcy. However, for some people, a more intensive intervention to help them to process the traumatic experience may be necessary before a person can even consider BA strategies.

Bringing it all together

Every encounter with a compassionate person is an opportunity for a traumatised individual to sow a seed towards enhanced self-care and empowerment. Even if some traumatised people speak and act in ways which practitioners find it difficult to warm to, thinking in a trauma-informed way can help us all to feel more skilled and to be more accepting. These ideas are equally applicable wherever we encounter traumatised people, from those who come often to the emergency department to those who rarely or reluctantly access support.

Tools for now: small changes that can make a big difference

It is essential when working with any patient, but particularly those who present with trauma-related complexities, that we notice how we are feeling and remain calm ourselves. Working in any health or care role requires managing our emotional load: if we do not feel calm, neither will our patients. Therefore, we can also use the Phase One techniques we teach our service users, such as paced breathing or grounding techniques, to help us manage our own emotions. It is important that we learn and practice using such tools before needing them and to enable us to promote them authentically. The ideas we share here are equally aimed to support the reader's own resilience and adaptive coping and are entirely in keeping with the relational 4 C's framework of TIC as described by Kimberg (2016): Calm, Contain, Care, and Cope. Every encounter with a health and social care professional is also an opportunity for positive experience in support of Phase Three: Reconnection.

Developing a battery of self-soothing strategies

Depending on your area of work, items may be made available for patients to use, such as small bottles of essential oil, stress balls, sensory objects or blankets. These are inexpensive, culturally neutral or diverse, can be calming and are linked to the environmental considerations of TIC. As in working with neurodiverse service users, paying attention to sensory and environmental sensitivities through a trauma-informed lens, can go a long way to easing distress and enabling resilience. Asking and working collaboratively to find the best available solution is even better. We may also need to ensure that we have additional time to offer the person with whom we are working, ensuring that we can manage the complexities of working with a trauma-lens. We hope that the evidence and resources referenced here will support the practitioner in their arguments to achieve this for their work area (Bulford et al., 2024).

Longer term approaches: supporting people to get 'Back to B.A.C.E.S.'

'Back to B.A.C.E.S.', BA is in keeping with factors that have been demonstrated to decrease vulnerability to the impact of complex trauma: firstly, by tapping into the individual's resilience (Ensink et al., 2020), secondly, by drawing attention to and mobilising resources and finally by mobilising valued relationships.

Body care

The health and social care practitioner may have extensive knowledge and resources to offer the traumatised individual around self-care, sleep, rest and relaxation, nutrition, hydration and exercise, but struggle to find a way in (Filson, 2016). We know that adverse childhood experiences (ACEs) are associated with negative health outcomes (Monnat and Chandler, 2015) and that this is likely to be mediated by maladaptive behaviours and their consequences, for example, emotional eating, alcohol and substance misuse for some, alongside poor sleep, poorer social attainment and social withdrawal. It follows that traumatised individuals, through maladaptive coping strategies, negative self-beliefs and social isolation, may not know about or practise basic self-care. Indeed, negative self-beliefs may make this seem counterintuitive, and they may not be in the habit of attending to their body and its needs (Monnat and Chandler, 2015).

Education, drawing attention to and offering encouragement towards Body and other self-care goals can be helpful and support a greater sense of routine and purpose, which in turn impacts positively on sleep and mood. A vast body of research now points to the importance of sleep for our physical and mental wellbeing and highly effective cognitive behavioural intervention programmes are available through the NHS and freely online to support better sleep (for example, the Sleepify App).

Achievement

When we think of achievement, we most often think in academic, financial or career terms. In the context of complex PTSD, re-engaging with such value-led factors may apply, but BA may begin with setting goals such as taking a shower, brushing one's teeth or returning a friend's call. Avoidance is a complicating factor for recovering from trauma and overcoming inactivity. People with complex trauma often withdraw from meaningful activities. Samaira's ability to settle into university life and make new friends was severely inhibited by her traumatised hyperarousal, manifesting as social anxiety and poor sleep. The loss of her focus on her studies once back home left more time for her to chew over trauma-related preoccupations, in turn leading to more intrusive memories of the abuse and negative self-talk. BA practically encourages disengagement with these unhelpful patterns and breaks the cycle of avoidance and isolation and lets in positive and rewarding experiences.

The principles of BA need to take account of the kind of sensitivities, which are common amongst traumatised people, by moving at a pace that accommodates hypervigilance, does not trigger dissociation or emotional flashbacks or interpersonal sensitivity. However, being listened to, invested in and having one's attention drawn to small gains can help with reinforcing positive change, as well as feelings of agency and control, which can become intrinsically motivating.

Regular engagement in valued activities can lead to improvement in mood, energy levels, and overall quality of life, addressing factors that make a person vulnerable to continuing complex PTSD.

Engaging in structured activities provides a sense of routine, purpose and positive reinforcement, which can improve mood instability. Samaira's catastrophic interpretation and location of trouble within herself was challenged by a conversation that helped her to articulate not just what was difficult about being at home, but what she could do to access more of the strategies that prompted adaptive coping, that she had acquired since leaving home. In addition to increased reminders of the adverse experiences she endured there and relationship challenges, she is without her university routine, friendships or the validating context of her studies and status as an undergraduate.

Connection

Complex trauma often damages relationships and trust so making time to connect with and invest in relationships with friends and family is an important aspect of recovery.

BA can reintroduce safe social interactions, helping individuals rebuild a sense of belonging and support. One consequence of Samaira's experience of sexual abuse was the negative impact on Samaira's peer relationships, which might otherwise have been protective of mental health in her adolescence (Wang et al., 2024). Samaira felt that she had to leave school early to protect her younger sister from the perpetrator. Aside from the impact on her education, this would have reduced opportunities for peer relationships and extracurricular opportunities supportive of self-esteem. Additionally, Samaira's comment about not feeling interest in the normative preoccupations of her peer group demonstrates her awareness of how her unique experience contributed to her social exclusion and development opportunities. Strong community ties and cultural connections are import-ant protective factors against the adverse effects of trauma.

Denial by caregivers of the reality of the individual's experience can be particularly damaging and impact on the person's relationships with others, beyond the family (Bolen and Lamb, 2007). We can see that for Samaira, another consequence of adverse experiences in childhood was her estrange-ment from her parents and siblings. Subsequent social isolation and lack of validation of the person's experience can lead to learned helplessness, thus increasing vulnerability to complex trauma and low mood (Crandall et al., 2024). By contrast, strong social connections are understood to serve as protective factors (Calhoun et al., 2022).

Enjoyment

This includes engaging in activities that are especially enjoyed and invit-ing fun in everyday life. Enhancing positive reinforcement – participating in enjoyable or meaningful activities – increases exposure to positive expe-riences that can counterbalance negative emotions stemming from trauma. Research about what sustains us, particularly in relation to self-care, motiva-tion and mood, emphasises systems of positive reinforcement and enjoying activities provides such reinforcement.

Spirituality

This may be religious practice or another form of more fundamental connec-tion with what matters to the person and their understanding of the bigger picture. One key element of Samaira's values is her faith. There have been a number of developments in adapting therapies to draw upon helpful aspects of faith beliefs, including Faith-Adapted BA (Mir et al., 2015, 2019, 2023). Samaira has an active faith and uses prayer to feel stronger. Compared to her relationships with friends and family, God has been an enduring and accepting presence throughout her life. Asking whether a person has faith-based beliefs to draw upon in troubled times is helpful in drawing their attention to their faith and conveying your own acceptance. For some people with strong religious beliefs or from a cultural background, which emphasises the importance of family loyalties, a person who has been sexually abused and disbelieved by parents, as Samaira has, may find themselves living with an overwhelmingly strong sense of guilt and community exclusion. Such a sense of guilt is not restricted to any one religious tradition or culture and is something to be aware of alongside positive aspects of faith and beliefs. Spirituality also encompasses values that link with an individual's morals, what matters and truly motivates them, enabling them to form a bridge with self-compassion. Pargament et al. (2000) have identified both positive and negative religious coping beliefs.

Summary of learning points

Within this chapter, we have reviewed a helpful framework for health and social care staff to consult when managing disclosure of traumatic experiences.

Enhanced personal resourcing for trauma survivors has been promoted and health and social care staff have been encouraged to see themselves as contributors to Phase One Trauma recovery.

BA literature has been explored and health and social care staff are encouraged to draw upon and strengthen existing skills within traumatised people who cross their path, through returning to the fundamentals of self-care in getting 'Back to B.A.C.E.S.' through the presentation of a newly adapted model for promoting self-care and wellbeing.

Questions for reflection and discussion

1. From what you know of Samaira's story and your own wider experience, what aspects of her developmental experience might still be working against her efforts to move on with her life?

2. What risks might exist around Samaira's emergency department visit that can act as a further disincentive for her to seek help and understanding?
3. What barriers to help-seeking might someone like Samaira face in the health or social care setting in which you work? Considering these, what might you do to overcome these or make their negative impact less likely?
4. How can you work to increase opportunities for promoting resilience, resourcing and relationship-building for people you work with, who may have experienced trauma.
5. In what ways could greater attention be paid to facilitating patients' and service users' recovery work around B.A.C.E.S. (Body and self-care, including sleep; Achievement through value led goals; Connections; Enjoyment and fun and Spirituality or meaning within your setting?

Recommended follow-up reading

Addis, M.E. and Martell, C.R. (2004). *Overcoming depression one step at a time: The new behavioral activation approach to getting your life back.* Oakland, CA: New Harbinger Pub.

Bar-Shai, M. and Klein, E. (2015). Vulnerability to PTSD: Psychosocial and demographic risk and resilience factors. In: Safir, M., Wallach, H., and Rizzo, A. (eds) *Future directions in post-traumatic stress disorder.* Boston, MA: Springer.

Every Mind Matters (n.d.). https://www.nhs.uk/every-mind-matters/mental-wellbeing-tips/how-to-fall-asleep-faster-and-sleep-better/ [Accessed 28th June 2025].

IICSA Independent Inquiry into Child Sexual Abuse, Reports Resources, https://www.iicsa.org.uk/reports-recommendations/publications/research.html [Accessed 28th June 2025].

NHS Wales University Health Board Psychological Therapies Department (n.d.). *An introduction to trauma: Stabilisation pack.* https://ctmuhb.nhs.wales/services/mental-health/self-help-resources/stabilisation-pack/stabilisation-pack/intro/an-introduction-to-trauma-pdf/ [Accessed 28th June 2025].

Trauma Research UK (n.d.). https://traumaresearchuk.org/the-54321-grounding-technique/ [Accessed 28th June 2025].

Notes

1   Hyperarousal is a key feature of post-traumatic reactions, impacting on relationships, sleep, cognitive abilities and physical health.
2   Emotional regulation is a term used to describe a person's ability to experience a wide range of emotions, to recognise them and to make links between their experience and mental or actual events and to call upon behavioural, or interpersonal strategies to re-establish equilibrium.

References

Baranowsky, A.B. and Gentry, J.E. (2015). *Trauma practice: Tools for stabilization and recovery*. Oxford and Boston: Hogrefe Publishing.

Bennice, J.A., Grubaugh, A.L. and Resick, P.A. (2001). Guilt, depression and PTSD among female rape victims. *Poster presented at the 17th Annual Meeting of the International Society for Traumatic Stress Studies*. New Orleans, USA.

Bolen, R.M. and Lamb, J.L. (2007). Parental support and outcome in sexually abused children. *Journal of Child Sexual Abuse*, 16(2): 33–54.

Brereton, A. and McGlinchey, E. (2019). Self-harm, emotion regulation, and experiential avoidance: A systematic review. *Archives of Suicide Research*, 24(sup1): 1–24.

Bulford, E., Baloch, S., Neil, J. and Hegarty, K. (2024). Primary healthcare practitioners' perspectives on trauma-informed primary care: A systematic review. *BMC Primary Care*, 25: 336.

Calhoun, C.D., Stone, K.J., Cobb, A.R., Patterson, M.W., Danielson, C.K. and Bendezú, J.J. (2022). The role of social support in coping with psychological trauma: An integrated biopsychosocial model for posttraumatic stress recovery. *Psychiatric Quarterly*, 93(4): 949–970.

Crandall, A., Castaneda, G.L., Barlow, M.J. and Magnusson, B.M. (2024). Do positive childhood and adult experiences counter the effects of adverse childhood experiences on learned helplessness? *Frontiers in Child and Adolescent Psychiatry*, 2: 12.

Dale, O., Sethi, F., Stanton, C., Evans, S., Barnicot, K., Sedgwick, R., Goldsack, S., Doran, M., Shoolbred, L., Samele, C., Urquia, N., Haigh, R. and Moran, P. (2017). Personality disorder services in England: Findings from a national survey. *BJPsych Bulletin*, 41(5): 247–253.

Department for Levelling Up, Housing and Communities (2023) *Trauma-informed approaches to supporting people experiencing multiple disadvantage: A rapid evidence assessment*. https://assets.publishing.service.gov.uk/media/642af3a77de 82b000c31350d/Changing_Futures_Evaluation_-_Trauma_informed_ approaches_REA.pdf [Accessed 27th May 2025].

Domhardt, M., Münzer, A., Fegert, J. and Goldbeck, L. (2015). Resilience in survivors of child sexual abuse. *Trauma Violence & Abuse*, 16: 476–493.

Ensink, K., Borelli, J.L., Normandin, L., Target, M. and Fonagy, P. (2020). Childhood sexual abuse and attachment insecurity: Associations with child psychological difficulties. *American Journal of Orthopedics*, 90: 115–124.

Etherton, J.L. and Farley, R. (2022). Behavioral activation for PTSD: A meta-analysis. *Psychol Trauma*, 14(5): 894–901.

Filson, B. (2016). The haunting can end: Trauma-informed approaches in healing from abuse and adversity. In Russo, J and Sweeney, A. (eds) *Searching for a rose garden: Challenging psychiatry, fostering mad studies 20–24*. Monmouth: PCCS Books.

Fok, M.L., Hayes, R.D., Chang, C.K., Stewart, R., Callard, F.J. and Moran, P. (2012). Life expectancy at birth and all-cause mortality among people with personality disorder. *Journal of Psychosomatic Research*, 73(2): 104–107.

Herman, J.L. (2022). *Trauma and recovery: The aftermath of violence – From domestic abuse to political terror* (Fourth trade paperback edition/with a new epilogue by the author.). New York: Basic Books.

Hunsaker, S., Chen, H.C., Maughan, D. and Heaston, S. (2015). Factors that influence the development of compassion fatigue, burnout, and compassion satisfaction in emergency department nurses. *Journal of Nursing Scholarship*, 47(2): 186–194.

Jakupcak, M. (2020). *The PTSD behavioral activation workbook: Activities to help you rebuild your life from post-traumatic stress disorder*. Oakland: New Harbinger Publications.

Johnstone, L., Boyle, M., with Cromby, J., Dillon, J., Harper, D., Kinderman, P., Longden, E., Pilgrim, D. and Read, J. (2018). *The power threat meaning framework: Towards the identification of patterns in emotional distress, unusual experiences and troubled or troubling behaviour, as an alternative to functional psychiatric diagnosis*. British Psychological Society. https://cms.bps.org.uk/sites/default/files/2022-07/PTM%20Framework%20%28January%202018%29_0.pdf [Accessed 28th June 2025].

Kanter, J.W., Santiago-Rivera, A.L., Santos, M.M., Nagy, G., López, M., Hurtado, G.D. and West, P. (2015). A randomized hybrid efficacy and effectiveness trial of behavioral activation for Latinos with depression. *Behavior Therapy*, 46(2): 177–192.

Kelly, L. and Todd, M. (2017). Compassion fatigue and the healthy work environment. *AACN Advanced Critical Care*, 28(4): 351–358.

Keyan, D., Garland, N., Choi-Christou, J., Tran, J., O'Donnell, M. and Bryant, R.A. (2024). A systematic review and meta-analysis of predictors of response to trauma-focused psychotherapy for posttraumatic stress disorder. *Psychological Bulletin*, 150(7): 767–797.

Kimberg, L. (2016). Trauma and trauma-informed care. In: King, T.E. and Wheeler M.B. (eds) *Medical management of vulnerable and underserved patients: Principles, practice, and populations* (2nd ed.), New York: McGraw-Hill.

Lamb, M.E., Brown, D.A., Hershkowitz, I., Orbach, Y. and Esplin, P.W. (2018). *Tell me what happened: Questioning children about abuse* (Wiley Series in Psychology of Crime, Policing and Law). Hoboken, NJ and Oxford: Wiley-Blackwell.

Lewis, C., Roberts, N.P., Gibson, S. and Bisson, J.I. (2020). Dropout from psychological therapies for post-traumatic stress disorder (PTSD) in adults: Systematic review and meta-analysis. *European Journal of Psychotraumatology*, 11(1): 1709709.

Mir, G., Ghani, R., Meer, S. and Hussain, G. (2019). Delivering a culturally adapted therapy for Muslim clients with depression. *Cognitive Behaviour Therapist*, 12: 1–14.

Mir, G., Meer, S., Cottrell, D., McMillan, D., House, A. and Kanter, J.W. (2015). Adapted behavioural activation for the treatment of depression in Muslims. *Journal of Affective Disorders*, 180: 190–199.

Mir, G., West, R., Meer, S., Rabbee, J. and Song, N. (2023). *Evaluating a culturally adapted behavioural activation therapy (BA-M)*. Leeds, UK: University of Leeds.

Monnat, S.M. and Chandler, R.F. (2015). Long term physical health consequences of adverse childhood experiences. *Sociol Q*, 56(4): 723–752.

Office for Health Improvement and Disparities (2022). *Working definition of trauma-informed practice*. https://www.gov.uk/government/publications/working-definition-of-trauma-informed-practice/working-definition-of-trauma-informed-practice#other-professional-resources-and-tools [Accessed 27th May 2025].

Ozer, E.J., Best, S.R., Lipsey, T.L. and Weiss, D.S. (2003). Predictors of posttraumatic stress disorder and symptoms in adults: A meta-analysis. *Psychological Bulletin*, 129(1): 52.

Pargament, K.I., Koenig, H.G. and Perez, L.M. (2000). The many methods of religious coping: Development and initial validation of the RCOPE. *Journal of Clinical Psychology*, 56(4): 519–543.

Read, A., Mazzucchelli, T.G. and Kane, R.T. (2016). A preliminary evaluation of a single session behavioural activation intervention to improve well-being and prevent depression in carers. *Clinical Psychologist*, 20(1): 36–45.

Reksoprodjo, M.R. (2023). Post traumatic growth inventory: Measuring the positive legacy of trauma on adolescences. *Journal of Advanced Education and Sciences*, 3(1): 97–101.

Resick, P.A. (2001). *Stress and trauma*. London: Psychology Press.

Rosenfield, P.J., Stratyner, A., Tufekcioglu, S., Karabell, S., McKelvey, J. and Litt, L. (2018). Complex PTSD in ICD-11: A case report on a new diagnosis. *Journal of Psychiatric Practice*, 24(5): 364–370.

Rushforth, A., Durk, M., Rothwell-Blake, G.A.A., Kirkman, A., Ng, F. and Kotera, Y. (2023). Self-compassion interventions to target secondary traumatic stress in healthcare workers: A systematic review. *International Journal of Environmental Research and Public Health*, 20(12): 6109.

Saunders, K.R.K., McGuinness, E., Barnett, P., Foye, U., Sears, J., Carlisle, S., Allman, F., Tzouvara, V., Schlief, M., Vera San Juan, N., Stuart, R., Griffiths, J., Appleton, R., McCrone, P., Rowan Olive, R., Nyikavaranda, P., Jeynes, T., K, T., Mitchell, L. and Simpson, A. (2023). A scoping review of trauma informed approaches in acute, crisis, emergency, and residential mental health care. *BMC Psychiatry*, 23(1): 1–36.

Sharp, S., Mcallister, M. and Broadbent, M. (2018). The tension between person centred and task focused care in an acute surgical setting: A critical ethnography. *Collegian*, 25(1): 11–17.

Stark, E. and Hester, M. (2019). Coercive control: Update and review. *Violence Against Women*, 25(1): 81–104.

Sweeney, A., Filson, B., Kennedy, A., Collinson, L. and Gillard, S. (2018). A paradigm shift: Relationships in trauma-informed mental health services. *BJPsych Advances*, 24(5): 319–333.

Wang, J.H., Merrin, G.J., Kiefer, S.M., Jackson, J.L., Huckaby, P.L., Pascarella, L.A., Blake, C.L., Gomez, M.D. and Smith, N.D.W. (2024). Peer relations of adolescents with adverse childhood experiences: A systematic literature review of two decades. *Adolescent Research Review*, 9(3): 477–512.

World Health Organisation (WHO) (2019). *International Classification of Diseases 11th Revision (ICD-11)*. https://www.who.int/standards/classifications/classification-of-diseases [Accessed 27th May 2025].

Zanarini, M.C., Gunderson, J.G., Marino, M.F., Schwartz, E.O. and Frankenburg, F.R. (1989). Childhood experiences of borderline patients. *Comprehensive Psychiatry*, 30(1): 18–25.

Health and care services and the risk of retraumatisation

Trudii Isherwood and
Lou Cherrill

Case study

Leigh's story

At 17 years old, I was admitted to a medical ward due to collapsing at home, believed to be due to my history of 'disordered eating' which had features of anorexia and bulimia, although this has never been diagnosed. I first saw mental health services when I was 13 and I self-harmed. This was my way of managing emotional and sexual abuse, seeing my parents abuse each other and misuse alcohol due to their mental ill-health, before they separated. They neglected me and bullied me due to my being bisexual which they were never able to accept. The bullying also happened at school, so I didn't attend much. I have social anxiety, am often depressed and anxious, and dissociate at times to manage how I feel.

After being admitted to hospital, I refused to eat. I was able to drink water, but I couldn't tolerate food, and I didn't want the nurses to give me an intravenous drip. I let them put in a naso-gastric feeding tube, but then it felt so strange I couldn't accept any food or supplements via the tube, and after three days, I got so frustrated I just pulled the tube out and wouldn't let them put another one in.

The people looking after me had a meeting and decided that I was a risk to myself because my physical health was getting worse, and that I needed to be put on a Section 3 of the Mental Health Act

DOI: 10.4324/9781003635604-7

so that they could legally force feed me. They tried to persuade me to eat, but in the end decided they had to restrain me to feed me. Some new nurses turned up who have special training in restraint, and they held me down on the bed while putting in a new feeding tube. I was held down for 30 minutes so that a feed could be given via the tube, and then, they took it out. I was so overwhelmed all I could do was lay there and blank them like it wasn't really happening to me. This happened every day for two weeks. I was meant to get mental health support, but because I was on a medical ward, this didn't always happen. My family were not interested, and they wouldn't visit me or support me. The staff also seemed upset by what they were doing to me, and I felt somewhat responsible for them being impacted by it. After two weeks, I decided enough was enough and I let them place the feeding tube and admit me to a specialist mental health unit. I ended up being there for a year, and we did work on the trauma of being restrained and force fed, and how this was retraumatising because of my history of being sexually abused. If they hadn't caused trauma and made my other traumas worse, I don't think I'd have been there for as long as I was.

Introduction

Trauma is not something that occurs independently in an individual, it is multilayered, dynamic, systemic and collective, having tremendous effects in all areas of health and wellbeing (Straussner and Calnan, 2014). As we see in Leigh's case study, the healthcare system can unintentionally traumatise or retraumatise people (Grossman et al., 2021). Trauma can also be caused by adverse childhood experiences (ACEs). As explained in earlier chapters, ACEs are stressful and negative events or situations, occurring in childhood or adolescence (Lorenc et al., 2020). An ACE can be a single event, or it can be repeated and prolonged events that effect emotions and behaviours, including the way a young person sees and interacts with their world (Senaratne et al., 2024). The trauma caused by ACEs have long-term consequences for physical and mental wellbeing (Senaratne et al., 2024).

Retraumatisation during contact with health services is not uncommon; however, services and staff often do not take this into account (Grossman et al., 2021). Those working in healthcare can also be traumatised and retraumatised or can be triggered and trigger the very people that they are trying to support. (See Chapter 9 for further information on the traumatised practitioner.)

Chapter aims

This chapter focuses on health and care services and the risk of retraumatisation and includes information and ideas related to:

- The retraumatising features of health and care services, both within specialist mental health provision and in health and care services more widely.
- The traumatising impact of dismissive attitudes and discrimination.
- Consideration of how the therapeutic relationship is impacted in the context of forced treatment.
- Understanding specialist interventions, including an exploration of specific issues around physical restraint in mental health services.

The retraumatising features of health and care services

Over half of all people will experience a trauma at some point in their lives (Brooks and Greenberg, 2024) so it follows that as a clinician, it will not be uncommon to encounter patients with some trauma history. While most people will experience only short-term distress as a result of a single trauma, for others, the trauma will impact all areas of the person and have a long-term effect on social, psychological and physical functioning (Brooks and Greenberg, 2024).

These experiences can affect trust and the way in which a person engages with family, friends and their world, including how they interact with and perceive health and care services. This applies particularly to the need to engage with health and care services in situations which can bring about uncomfortable experiences and mixed emotions (Harricharan et al., 2021).

On a system level, much is reported in the media about the perceived failings of the NHS, with 24% of people in England reporting an experience of poor care (Kennedy, 2025). Headlines include stories of babies dying due to hostile ward cultures, inability to access emergency care and the many documented horrors of the COVID-19 pandemic. It would not be surprising that people without an existing trauma would feel anxious trusting their wellbeing to a struggling system. The impact of media exposure on anxiety in relation to COVID-19 has been explored in research (Greenhawt et al., 2021). Expectant mothers left waiting for hours for scans may wonder whether the same lack of attention may happen during delivery. Similarly, a worried son who heard how people died alone during the pandemic, may feel overwhelmed with anxiety when told that he cannot visit his seriously ill parent due to a Norovirus outbreak.

For those who have experienced trauma, intense feelings can swiftly be reignited by an unintentional thoughtless or detrimental experience such as not recognising that sexual assault victims may need additional support during intimate examinations (Grossman et al., 2021). Consider first, the familiar apprehension felt by many women when attending their local doctor's surgery for a smear test. Then, think of the same experience from the viewpoint of a victim of sexual assault. The dichotomy of needing to protect oneself against a potential cancer versus the possibility of reliving an experience of personal violation is easily recognisable (Widanaralalage et al., 2024).

It is common for people to feel devoid of control when attending healthcare appointments alongside feeling that by opening up to the expertise of the professionals, we are laying aside our own autonomy. A procedure which may feel like a routine day-to-day activity to the health practitioner – including the removal of clothing, physical touch or the giving of bad news – is in no way routine for the person on the receiving end (Devillers et al., 2023). The balance of power sits with the professional, and it can feel unnervingly disempowering to temporarily surrender the norms of everyday social interactions to the point of undressing in front of a stranger, even in the context of the most positive of interactions (Devillers et al., 2023). Add into this a trauma history, where these seemingly routine procedures can trigger a traumatic memory, and it is unsurprising that engaging with health and care services can cause harm to occur or resurface (Huo et al., 2023).

This is applicable to all health and care services, although is more profound within mental health inpatient services, both because of the nature of the care environment and because of the higher prevalence of existing trauma within this patient group (Saunders et al., 2023). While trauma is not caused by mental illness, much mental illness is caused by trauma. Indeed, some authorities have suggested that all mental ill-health might be caused by trauma (Dye, 2018). Thus, there is potential for an ongoing pattern of trauma and retraumatisation, with health and care sitting within and perpetuating the cycle (Hennessy et al., 2022).

Mental health wards are supposed to be a safe haven and a place to recover, but the reality for many people is that the experience of admission to a mental health setting causes trauma to resurface (Hennessy et al., 2022). Much has been written about upsetting and distressing experiences in mental health settings, ranging from intractable boredom to restrictive practices, which include intrusive observations (such as when showering, bathing or using the toilet), seclusion and restraint, all taking place in poor physical environments, where social interactions and lack of choice lead to feelings of infantilisation and exclusion from any activity that enhances a sense of self-efficacy (Hennessy et al., 2022). Both research and autobiographical literature describe patients feeling traumatised by their experiences of contact with mental health services (Sweeney et al., 2018).

It is common to respond to patient distress by trying to shut it down, with emotional suppression being a method of emotional regulation (Thuillard and Dan-Glauser, 2020). Fortunately, the use of restrictive interventions is now less common, although the routine chemical management of emotional distress is the norm in mental health services and beyond (Min and Alemi, 2025). While psychiatric medications can have a valuable place in supporting recovery from mental ill health, there is a risk that this internalises the issue (Sharma-Patel and Brown, 2016) by suggesting that although someone or something has traumatised you, you need a pill to rebalance your brain. The implication, therefore, is that you are the problem, and the issue lies with you. When this intervention is forced, via intramuscular injections whilst detained under a Section of the Mental Health Act, the potential for self-blame and retraumatisation escalates enormously.

Eating is clearly a physical need, as we cannot exist without adequate nutrition, but there are many interlinked social and psychological constructs linked to the act of taking (and not taking) food (Dakin et al., 2024). A person detained under the Mental Health Act (1983) can be force fed if it is felt that the action is necessary to treat their underlying mental illness. However, forced feeding is an extraordinarily complex issue, fraught with emotional and ethical considerations (Ruck Keene 2019). The link between food and mental health and wellbeing (Firth et al., 2020) has been acknowledged throughout history. In the 19th century, the refusal to eat was seen as a sign of insanity, and something that needed to be managed with physical force (van Deth and Vandereycken, 2000). Force-feeding prisoners on hunger strike has been likened to an experience worse than rape (Miller, 2016).

Eating disorders often manifest in times of chaos to foster a sense of order within the individual. Psychologically, they can create a sense of control over the person's own body in an internal and external world where there is little control over anything else (Frolich et al., 2020). There is undoubtedly a link between sexual abuse and the loss of body autonomy that this brings about, with a higher-than-average rate of eating disorders being seen in survivors of sexual abuse (Kimber et al., 2017). Taking this control away can be devastating and highly retraumatising. Hospital admission per se, even when not under duress and for a simple physical procedure, can be viewed by a patient as losing their fundamental right to choice and bodily autonomy. There can be a loss of usual routine, restrictions on seeing family and friends, as well as lack of choice over food and drinks, to name a few.

If layered on top of this is the removal of an area of control that is an ingrained and robust coping mechanism and therefore a protective factor, by way of a legal restriction and physical curtailment, it is not surprising that existing trauma will be relived, and new trauma established on top of this, regardless of professional and legal arguments stating that the forced feeding interventions are used to preserve life (Frolich et al., 2020).

While there is no single cause for an eating disorder it can often be a build-up of stressful experiences, including, as for Leigh, neglect and abuse. Leigh's neglect was multifaceted but included being without sufficient nutrition, both due to poverty and caregiver failings. Their disordered eating had both a cause-and-effect relationship with this experience, but there would have been a complex retraumatisation resulting from force feeding and the decision for their family to distance themselves from it.

By the time Leigh had been admitted to hospital, they had experienced many years of contact with a range of professionals. A number of these contacts had not been positive, and each time Leigh was transferred or moved between teams, the feelings of abandonment from childhood were triggered until they got to the point where they were unable to positively engage at all. At the same time, their physical health deteriorated so much that a hospital admission became unavoidable.

Compounding the admission was the fact that starvation was only worsening Leigh's mental health, which was then making it even harder to eat. Leigh had also been living for a long time in a state of chronic stress, which is itself linked to poor health outcomes (Seib et al., 2014). It has been found that a higher number of ACEs can be an indicator of poor physical health (Senaratne et al., 2024). Trauma can manifest physically in the form of flashbacks, or with the release of stress hormones, as well as with a continual retriggering of the fight or flight response (Dye, 2018).

The field of epigenetics explores how experience and stress shapes DNA, and while the exact mechanism is unknown, chronic stress can be passed through generations (Nestler, 2016). Leigh's direct family had a history of mental illness and alcohol abuse long before Leigh was born, which may have contributed to Leigh's predisposition (Ning et al., 2020).

All of this meant that the person being admitted for physical collapse had a lot of undiagnosed and unmanaged trauma, and while this had been recognised, the primary focus has become Leigh's physical health. As much as nobody set out to ignore their mental health issues, their life was at the point of being at risk if they did not take some nutrition. Unfortunately, this led to physical restraint and forced feeding.

The traumatising impact of dismissive attitudes

It is not uncommon for trauma survivors to find their experiences are denied by family, their communities and society, and even by institutions that purportedly exist to support people in this position. This concept, known as 'unvictiming' (Watts, 2024) can be in the form of direct disbelief, minimising or dismissing the experience or its impact, to going as far as the direct or subtle blaming of the victim for what has happened to them.

Where trauma is linked to mental illness, there is an added layer of stigma (Walsh and Foster, 2024). Although there are claims that the stigma around mental illness has reduced in recent years, around 90% of people with mental health-related diagnoses still report that the stigma of being mentally unwell has negatively affected them (Mental Health Foundation, 2021).

Dismissive behaviour can range from indifference to disrespect to direct rudeness, and it may seem perverse that dismissive behaviour can itself be caused by trauma and be a protective mechanism against low self-esteem and an inability to cope with conflict (Dabekaussen et al., 2023). Dismissive behaviour that perpetuates stigma is displayed at more than an individual level. Structural stigma is defined as the *'societal-level conditions, cultural norms, and institutional policies that constrain the opportunities, resources, and wellbeing of the stigmatized'* (Hatzenbuehler, 2016: 1).

Marginalised groups often face more dismissive attitudes to their trauma with contact with institutions, including health and social care organisations and services (Skosireva et al., 2014). Lesbian, gay, bisexual, transgender, queer, questioning, or intersex communities, along with others not identifying as cisgender or hetero-normative (LGBTQIA+), can experience challenges such as isolation and marginalisation, which can lead to a higher number of ACEs (Wilson and Cariola, 2020). They therefore have more existing experiences of trauma as they enter into a system that often rejects them (Stein et al., 2023). Women who have experienced trauma are more likely to be given a diagnosis of a personality disorder (Swart et al., 2020). In these and other ways, society continues to send the message to the traumatised individual that they are at fault for their trauma (Watts, 2024).

When healthcare professionals can reflect on and recognise the detrimental impact of dismissive attitudes and stigma, this can be the catalyst for a profound shift in the direction of providing trauma-informed services. Understanding that dismissive behaviour can retraumatise individuals, professionals can become more empathic, validating patients' experiences and creating an environment of trust (Yu et al., 2022).

The impact of forced treatment on the therapeutic relationship

Physical restraint and forced feeding have a traumatic impact on Leigh, with part of this impact being the complete fracturing of the relationship between them and the clinical teams who were part of the intervention (Ebun, 2023).

Leigh had not had secure and positive attachments and relationships for most of their life. These ACEs could have triggered mental health problems, as ACEs have been shown to effect perception of others' attitudes about the self, via the impact of depression (Salokangas et al., 2018). Leigh found trust difficult and brought that trauma to a situation where 'caregivers', in

Leigh's eyes, removed their dignity and choice over every aspect of their being. The effect on them was devastating and took a long time to begin to come to terms with.

Therapeutic relationships are difficult to establish and maintain in restrictive and forced interventions (Ebun, 2023). Indeed, historically, the 'response' teams who dealt with these incidents were often people not known to the patients in order that the 'therapy' team could maintain a connection. However, this increases issues of strangers putting hands on the person, which is likely to be even more traumatising (Care Quality Commission, 2024).

A patient and therapist will both bring their history to a relationship, and this introduces issues relating to transference influencing interactions between them (Hughes and Kerr, 2018). The patient will often bring a trauma history as well, and trust and mutual respect are needed to prevent retraumatisation. The utter violation experienced by patients who have been given forced treatment can make it challenging to form and maintain relationships. It is therefore imperative that health practitioners respond in a trauma-informed manner (Ebun, 2023).

It is also vital to recognise that trauma affects everyone, and therefore, staff may bring their own trauma to work and be retraumatised whilst just doing their job. This trauma can be personal or indeed experienced at work and reinforced at work. Supervision and support are critical components for healthcare professionals to effectively manage the impacts of vicarious trauma.

Tools for now: small changes that can make a big difference

Supporting steps to recovery

- Adopt a holistic approach, acknowledging the full spectrum of a patient's trauma history and its influence on their mental and physical health.
- Confront and reduce stigma, seeking to create a more inclusive and supportive healthcare environment which empowers patients, to improve therapeutic outcomes and promote healing (Song et al., 2023).
- A paradigm shift, from judgement to understanding, not only benefits individual patient care but also advances the overarching goal of equitable and compassionate healthcare for all.

Taking care of yourself

Health and care professionals working within mental health settings with patients experiencing mental distress and trauma are very likely to encounter emotionally charged situations and upsetting patient narratives, which can lead to vicarious trauma whereby individuals experience trauma symptoms due to exposure to another person's traumatic experiences (Branson, 2019). Regular supervision provides a structured environment where healthcare workers can reflect on their emotional responses, gain insights, and develop coping strategies (Rothwell et al., 2021). Support from peers and supervisors fosters a sense of community and shared understanding, mitigating feelings of isolation. This collective approach enhances resilience, ensuring healthcare professionals maintain their wellbeing and continue providing compassionate care. Prioritising supervision and support not only benefit individual practitioners but also contribute to a healthier, more sustainable healthcare system (HCPC, 2021).

Trauma-informed care in everyday healthcare practice

Working in a trauma-informed way does not mean treating the trauma. It means to heed and be mindful of the issues that survivors have when accessing health and care to prevent retraumatisation. Applying the key principles of trauma-informed practice (Office for Health Improvement and Disparities, 2022) to the example previously mentioned of a sexual assault victim attending for a smear test helps to illustrate the importance of trauma-informed care in everyday healthcare practice.

Safety is both physical and psychological. It should include the immediate environment of healthcare delivery as well as the policy and guidance shaping service delivery (Grailey et al., 2021). All too often smear tests are done after half an hour in a busy and loud waiting room, with no time to adjust psychologically and emotionally before taking off clothes behind flimsy curtains which afford little in the way of feelings of privacy. There is not always the opportunity for a personal chaperone. Potential ways of promoting safety include offering more information in the appointment letter, offering the test in a different location such as a women's centre, and suggesting that the woman brings someone of their choice along with them.

Distrust can be an outcome of past trauma (Bell et al., 2018), making it more difficult to foster trust with someone you may only meet every 5 years for this intimate examination. While trauma survivors may not be able to trust their professionals, that does not mean we should not strive to be trust-worthy, both individually and systemwide (Varga et al., 2023).

Giving choice can be hard within an under-resourced system but small changes can make a huge difference to trauma survivors. Co-creating health and social care services in partnership with service users can increase choice and collaboration into all healthcare interactions (Halvorsrud et al., 2021). The resulting empowerment can be validating and give power to a person who feels powerless. Additional effort should be taken when addressing trauma for minority groups, and people whose voices are not always heard.

The validation created by adopting trauma-informed practices can empower a sexual abuse victim to proactively engage with services both for themselves and to help others. To suggest words and positions that are less likely to be distressing, to have music and headphones on, to offer pre-appointments where everything can be explained, are small changes that can be made without any disclosure from the patient. A less frightening and more empow-ering experience can reduce the fear, building on recovery over time.

Trauma causes invalidation, fear, hypervigilance and shame. Often the 'system' plays a part in the trauma, yet it is this same system to which peo-ple need to turn for support with recovery. It is therefore vital that we do all that is possible to shape services in ways which avoid retraumatisation. Unfortunately, some interventions are at times deemed necessary to prevent serious harm. Recognising how these can mimic the original trauma as well as taking away coping mechanisms and retraumatising, are essential aspects of validating and mitigating the subsequent distress and distrust of service providers (Grailey et al., 2021).

Understanding specialist interventions: physical restraint

Restrictive interventions are defined by the Department of Health (DoH) as 'deliberate acts on the part of other person(s) that restrict an individual's movement, liberty and/or freedom to act independently' (DoH, 2014: 14). The DoH guidance on Positive and Proactive Care: reducing the need for restrictive interventions (2014) acknowledges that in mental health care, it has been the case historically that physical interventions have been used to punish and humiliate and that they generally delay recovery. There is also an acknowledgement that they can cause physical and psychological trauma to patients and staff. Restrictive interventions are now less used, although it is argued that there is a need for physical or chemical restraint where the patient or others are at immediate risk of serious harm.

Restrictive interventions are permitted under the Mental Health Act (1983) and under common law where there is an urgent necessity. Nonetheless, even though the use of restrictive interventions is deemed legal in some circumstances, these practices evoke considerable debate around human rights (Equality and Human Rights Commission, 2019).

It has been discussed that simply being a patient can be a situation where control and choice is already lacking and there is risk of reliving traumatic events. While this is mostly unintentional and many healthcare staff will do their utmost to empower the patient as much as possible as an active participant in decision making, the potential for compounding psychological harm is nonetheless real in these settings.

Restraint, however, is deliberate and intended. While there are reports that restraint can help a person in crisis feel safe, there are also reports of unnecessary practice, exacerbated by a restrictive environment (Hammervold et al., 2019). Even if the restraint is evaluated as being justified and necessary as a last resort, the trauma does not lessen for those on the receiving end.

There are higher than average rates of physical and sexual abuse to be found in mental health patients (Khalifeh et al., 2016), making restrictive interventions, and particularly restraint more profoundly damaging. Being restrained can make a person feel helpless and humiliated (Wong et al., 2020), feelings which resound echoes of some trauma situations. It can trigger a pattern in poor coping mechanisms, increasing aggression and causing post-traumatic stress disorder (PTSD) as well as interrupting and destroying the potential for therapeutic relationships, which in turn compounds difficulties with debriefing (Price et al., 2024). Restraint also produces physical trauma to an already fragile physiological state of a person weakened by chronic stress and hypervigilance. Furthermore, the experience can trigger an acute stress response, and the need for fight-or-flight in a situation where there is no escape.

Leigh experienced both forced feeding and physical restraint. The simple act of being hospitalised is traumatising, but Leigh is in hospital against their will, in a fragile physical state and with a complex trauma history. Every part of their time on the ward would be likely to have retraumatised them in extremely complex and interdependent ways. It is not surprising that they spent such a long time in a specialist placement afterwards. The alternative, however, would have been to risk letting them starve, and this is clearly not something that was legal or ethical.

Summary of learning points

This chapter has explored a range of theoretical and practical approaches to understanding and managing the risks of retraumatisation in health and care settings, including:

- The understanding that trauma impacts everyone and recognition that acknowledging this is a key aspect of improving patient care and staff wellbeing.
- Even with the most beneficent intentions, health and care services can both cause and reignite trauma. Providing quality services requires an awareness of this throughout the healthcare team, alongside a willingness and determination to create a culture that does not retraumatise.
- Where this is not possible, in situations where someone's life is at risk, we must acknowledge the impact on service users and patients, doing all we can to support the person to understand why what has happened took place, and to help them on their journey to recovery.

Questions for reflection and discussion

1. Using the six key principles of trauma-informed practice (safety, trust, choice, collaboration, empowerment and cultural consider- ations), reflect upon whether any of these principles were consid- ered for Leigh. If not, why not?
2. What could have been done differently to support Leigh to recover and potentially avoid the exacerbation of trauma before, during and after their experience of hospital admission?

3. Has thinking about Leigh's experience changed how you will approach your future practice, and if yes, how? Which of the six principles of trauma-informed care can you most easily implement in your day-to-day practice?
4. How can you offer holistic care to service users and patients who have been retraumatised by their previous experiences in health and care situations?
5. What steps can you take to raise awareness of retraumatisation in health and care situations amongst colleagues?

Recommended follow-up reading

Office for Health Improvement and Disparities. (2022). *Working definition of trauma-informed practice*. GOV.UK. https://www.gov.uk/government/publications/working-definition-of-trauma-informed-practice [Accessed 29th May 2025].

SAMHSA. (2014). *SAMHSA's concept of trauma and guidance for a trauma-informed approach*. SAMHSA Publications and Digital Products. https://library.samhsa.gov/sites/default/files/sma14-4884.pdf [Accessed 29th May 2025].

Department of Health. (2014). *Positive and proactive care: Reducing the need for restrictive interventions*. https://assets.publishing.service.gov.uk/media/5a7ee560e5274a2e8ab48e2a/JRA_DoH_Guidance_on_RP_web_accessible.pdf [Accessed 29th May 2025].

Equality and Human Rights Commission. (2019). *Human rights framework for restraint*. https://www.equalityhumanrights.com/sites/default/files/human-rights-framework-restraint.pdf [Accessed 29th May 2025].

References

Bell, V., Robinson, B., Katona, C., Fett, A.K. and Shergill, S. (2018). When trust is lost: The impact of interpersonal trauma on social interactions. *Psychological Medicine*, 49(6): 1041–1046.

Branson, D.C. (2019). Vicarious trauma, themes in research, and terminology: A review of literature. *Traumatology*, 25(1): 2–10.

Brooks, S.K. and Greenberg, N. (2024). Recurrence of post-traumatic stress disorder: Systematic review of definitions, prevalence and predictors. *BMC Psychiatry*, 24: 37.

Care Quality Commission. (2024). *Restrictive practices*. https://www.cqc.org.uk/publications/monitoring-mental-health-act/2022-2023/restrictive-practices?form=MG0AV3 [Accessed 8th February 2025].

Dabekaussen, K.F.A.A., Scheepers, R.A., Heineman, E., Haber, A.L., Lombarts, K.M.J.M.H., Jaarsma, D.A.D.C. and Shapiro, J. (2023). Health care professionals' perceptions of unprofessional behaviour in the clinical workplace. *PLOS One.* 18(1):1–14.

Dakin, C., Finlayson, G. and Stubbs, R.J. (2024). Exploring the underlying psychological constructs of self-report eating behavior measurements: Towards a comprehensive framework. *Psychological Review.* Advance online publication.

Department of Health. (2014). *Positive and proactive care: Reducing the need for restrictive interventions.* https://assets.publishing.service.gov.uk/media/5a7ee560e5274a2e8ab48e2a/JRA_DoH_Guidance_on_RP_web_accessible.pdf [Accessed 29th May 2025].

Devillers, L., Subts, A., De Bandt, D., Druais, P.L. and de la, L. (2023). Patients' experiences of being touched by their general practitioner: A qualitative study. *British Medical Journal Open*, 13: e071701.

Dye, H. (2018). The impact and long-term effects of childhood trauma. *Journal of Human Behaviour in the Social Environment*, 28(3): 381–392.

Ebun, T.J. (2023). Women's experiences of restrictive interventions in inpatient units and how they impact their recovery. *Cognizance Journal of Multidisciplinary Studies*, 3(10): 140–173.

Equality and Human Rights Commission. (2019). *Human rights framework for restraint: Principles for the lawful use of physical, chemical, mechanical and coercive restrictive interventions.* https://www.equalityhumanrights.com/sites/default/files/human-rights-framework-restraint.pdf [Accessed 29th May 2025].

Firth, J., Gangwisch, J.E., Borsini, A., Wootton, R.E. and Mayer, E.A. (2020). Food and mood: How do diet and nutrition affect mental wellbeing? *The British Medical Journal*, 369: m2382.

Frolich, J., Winkler, L.A.D., Abrahamsen, B., Bilenberg, N., Hermann, A.P. and Stoving, R.K. (2020). Assessment of fracture risk in women with eating disorders: The utility of dual-energy x-ray absorptiometry (DXA) – Clinical cohort studies. *International Journal of Eating Disorders*, 53(4): 595–605.

Grailey, K.E., Murray, E., Reader, T. and Brett, S.J. (2021). The presence And potential impact of psychological safety in the healthcare setting: An evidence synthesis. *BMC Health Services Research*, 21: 773.

Greenhawt, M., Kimball, S., DunnGalvin, A., Abrams, E.M., Shaker, M.S., Mosnaim, G., Comberiati, P., Nekliudov, N.A., Blyuss, O., Teufel, M. and Munblit, D. (2021). Media influence on anxiety, health utility, and health beliefs early in the SARS-Cov-2 pandemic – A survey study. *Journal of General Internal Medicine*, 36: 1327–1337.

Grossman, S., Cooper, Z., Buxton, H., Hendrickson, S., Lewis, -, O'Connor, A., Stevens, J., Wong, L.Y. and Bonne, S. (2021). Trauma-informed care: Recognizing and resisting re-traumatization in health care. *Trauma Surgery & Acute Care Open*, 6(1): 1–5.

Halvorsrud, K., Kucharska, J., Adlington, K., Rudell, K., Hajdukova, E.B., Nazroo, J., Haarmans, M., Rhodes, J. and Bhui, K. (2021). Identifying evidence of effectiveness in the co-creation of research: A systematic review and meta-analysis of the international healthcare literature. *Journal of Public Health*, 41(1): 197–208.

Hammervold, U.E., Norvoll, R., Aas, R.W. and Sagvaag, H. (2019). Post-incident review after restraint in mental health care – A potential for knowledge development, recovery promotion and restraint prevention. A scoping review. *BMC Health Services Research*, 19: 235.

Harricharan, S., McKinnon, M. and Lanius, R.A. (2021). How processing of sensory information from the internal and external worlds shape the perception and engagement with the world in the aftermath of trauma: Implications for PTSD. *Frontiers in Neuroscience*, 15: 1–20.

Hatzenbuehler, M.L. (2016). Structural stigma: Research evidence and implications for psychological science. *American Psychologist*, 71(8): 742–751.

HCPC. (2021). *The benefits and outcomes of effective supervision*. https://www.hcpc-uk.org/standards/meeting-our-standards/supervision-leadership-and-culture/supervision/the-benefits-and-outcomes-of-effective-supervision/ [Accessed 8th February 2025].

Hennessy, B., Hunter, A. and Grealish, A. (2022). A qualitative synthesis of patients' experiences of re-traumatisation in acute mental health inpatient settings. *Journal of Psychiatric and Mental Health Nursing*, 30: 398–434.

Hughes, P. and Kerr, I. (2018). Transference and countertransference in communication between doctor and patient. *Advances in Psychiatric Treatment*, 6(1): 57–64.

Huo, Y., Couzner, L., Windsor, T., Laver, K., Dissanayaka, N.N. and Cations, M. (2023). Barriers and enablers for the implementation of trauma-informed care in healthcare settings: A systematic review. *Implementation Science Communications*, 4: 49.

Kennedy, B. (2025). Serious failings in NHS complaints system leaves patients reluctant to speak out, says patient watch dog. *The British Medical Journal*, 388: r180.

Khalifeh, H., Oram, S., Osborn, D., Howard, L.M. and Johnson, S. (2016). Recent physical and sexual violence against adults with severe mental illness: A systematic review and meta-analysis. *International Review of Psychiatry*, 28(5): 433–451.

Kimber, M., McTavish, J.R., Couturier, J., Boven, A., Gill, S., Dimitropoulos, G. and MacMillan, H.L. (2017). Consequences of child emotional abuse, emotional neglect and exposure to intimate partner violence for eating disorders: A systematic critical review. *BMC Psychology*, 5: 33.

Lorenc, T., Lester, S., Sutcliffe, K., Stansfield, C. and Thomas, J. (2020). Interventions to support people exposed to adverse childhood experiences: Systematic review of systematic reviews. *BMC Public Health*, 20: 657.

Mental Health Act. (1983). https://www.legislation.gov.uk/ukpga/1983/20/contents?-form=MG0AV3 [Accessed 8th February 2025].

Mental Health Foundation. (2021). Stigma and discrimination. https://www.mentalhealth.org.uk/explore-mental-health/a-z-topics/stigma-and-discrimination [Accessed 8th February 2025].

Miller, I. (2016). *A history of force feeding: Hunger strikes, prisons and medical ethics, 1909-1974*. Basingstoke: Palgrave Macmillan.

Min, H. and Alemi, F. (2025). Insights into prescribing practices for antidepressants: An evidence-based analysis. *BMC Medical Informatics and Decision Making*, 25(1): 42.

Nestler, E.J. (2016). Transgenerational epigenetic contributions to stress responses: Fact or fiction? *PLoS Biology*, 14(3): 1–7.

Ning, K., Gondek, D., Patalay, P. and Ploubidis, G.B. (2020). The association between early life mental health and alcohol use behaviours in adulthood: A systematic review. *PLOS One*. 15(2): 1–28.

Office for Health Improvement and Disparities. (2022). *Working definition of trauma-informed practice*. GOV.UK https://www.gov.uk/government/publications/working-definition-of-trauma-informed-practice [Accessed 29th May 2025].

Price, O., Armitage, C.J., Bee, P., Brooks, H., Lovell, K., Butler, D., Cree, L., Fishwick, P., Grundy, A., Johnston, I., Mcpherson, P., Riches, H., Scott, A., Walker, L. and Brooks, C.P. (2024). De-escalating aggression in acute inpatient mental health settings: A behaviour change theory-informed, secondary qualitative analysis of staff and patient perspectives. *BMC Psychiatry*, 24: 548.

Ruck Keene,, A. (2019). *The MHA, force-feeding and best interests*. https://www.mentalcapacitylawandpolicy.org.uk/the-mha-force-feeding-and-best-interests/ [Accessed 29th May 2025].

Rothwell, C., Kehoe, A., Farook, S.F. and Illing, J. (2021). Enablers and barriers to effective clinical supervision in the workplace: A rapid evidence review. *BMJ Open*, 11: e052929.

Salokangas, R.K.R., From, T., Luutonen, S. and Heitala, J. (2018). Adverse childhood experiences leads to perceived negative attitude of others and the effect of adverse childhood experiences on depression in adulthood is mediated via negative attitude of others. *European Psychiatry*, 54: 27–34.

Saunders, K.R.K., McGuinness, E., Barnett, P., Foye, U., Sears, J., Carlisle, S., Allman, F., Tzouvara, V., Schlief, M., Juan, N.V.S., Stuart, R., Griffiths, J., Appleton, R., McCrone, P., Oliver, R.R., Nyikavaranda, P., Tamar Jeynes, T.K., Mitchall, M., Simpson, A., Johnson, S. and Trevillion, K. (2023). A scoping review of trauma informed approaches in acute, crisis, emergency, and residential mental health care. *BMC Psychiatry*, 23, 567.

Seib, C., Whiteside, E., Humphreys, J., Lee, K., Thomas, P., Chopin, L., Crisp, G., O'Keeffe, A., Kimlin, M., Stacey, A. and Anderson, D. (2014). A longitudinal study of the impact of chronic psychological stress on health-related quality of life and clinical biomarkers: Protocol for the Australian healthy aging of women study. *BMC Public Health*, 14: 9.

Senaratne, D.N.S., Thakkar, B., Smith, B.H., Hales, T.G., Marryat, L. and Colvin, L.A. (2024). The impact of adverse childhood experiences on multimorbidity: A systematic review and meta-analysis. *BMC Medicine*, 22: 315.

Sharma-Patel, K. and Brown, E.J. (2016). Emotion regulation and self blame as mediators and moderators of trauma-specific treatment. *Psychology of Violence*, 6(3): 400–409.

Skosireva, A., O'Campo, P., Zerger, S., Chambers, C., Gapka, S. and Stergiopoulos, V. (2014). Different faces of discrimination: Perceived discrimination among homeless adults with mental illness in healthcare settings. *BMC Health Services Research*, 14: 376.

Song, N., Hugh-Jones, S., West, R.M., Pickavance, J. and Mir, G. (2023). The effectiveness of anti-stigma interventions for reducing mental health stigma in young people: A systematic review and meta-analysis. *Cambridge Prisms: Global Mental Health*, 10: e39.

Stein, G.L., Berkman, C., Acquaviva, K., Woody, I., Godfrey, D., Javier, N.M., O'Mahony, S., Gonzalex-Rivera, C., Maingi, S., Candrian, C. and Rosa, W.E. (2023). Project respect: Experiences of seriously ill LGBTQ+ patients and partners with their health providers. *Health Affairs Scholar*, 1(4): 1–9.

Straussner, S.L.A. and Calnan, A.J. (2014). Trauma through the life cycle: A review of current literature. *Clinical Social Work Journal*, 42: 323–335.

Swart, S., Wildschut, M., Draijer, N., Langeland, W., Hoogendoorn, A.W. and Smit, J.H. (2020). The course of (comorbid) trauma-related, dissociative and personality disorders: Two year follow up of the Friesland study cohort. *European Journal of Psychotraumatology*, 11(1): 1–11.

Sweeney, A., Filson, B., Kennedy, A., Collison, L. and Gillard, S. (2018). A paradigm shift: Relationships in trauma-informed mental health services. *BJPsych Advances*, 24(5): 319–333.

Thuillard, S. and Dan-Glauser, E.S. (2020). The simultaneous use of *emotional suppression* and *situation selection* to regulate emotions incrementally favors physiological responses. *BMC Psychology*, 8: 133.

van Deth, R. and Vandereycken, W. (2000). Food refusal and insanity: Sitophobia and anorexia nervosa in Victorian asylums. *The International Journal of Eating Disorders*, 27(4): 390–404.

Varga, A.I., Spehar, I. and Skirbekk, H. (2023). Trustworthy management in hospital settings: A systematic review. *BMC Health Services Research*, 23: 662.

Walsh, D. and Foster, J. (2024). Understanding the public stigma of mental illness: A mixed-methods, multi-level, exploratory triangulation study. *BMC Psychology*, 12: 403.

Watts, J. (2024). Complex trauma and the unseen: Who gets to be a victim? *BMJ Mental Health*, 27: e301240.

Widanaralalage, B.K., Murphy, A.D. and Loughlin, C. (2024). Support or justice: A triangulated multi-focal view of sexual assault victim support in a UK sexual assault referral centre (SARC). *International Journal of Mental Health Systems*, 18: 15.

Wilson, C. and Cariola, L.A. (2020). LGBTQI+ youth and mental health: A systematic review of qualitative research. *Adolescent Research Review*, 5: 187–211.

Wong, A.H., Ray, J.M., Rosenberg, A., Crispino, L., Parker, J., McVaney, C., BS, Lennaco, J.D., Bernstein, S.L. and Pavlo, A.J. (2020). Experiences of individuals who were physically restrained in the emergency department. *JAMA Network Open*, 3(1): e1919381.

Yu, C.C., Tan, L., Le, M.K., Tang, B., Liaw, S.Y., Tierney, T., Ho, Y.Y., Lim, B.E.E., Lim, D., NG, R., Chia, S.C. and Low, J.A. (2022). The development of empathy in the healthcare setting: A qualitative approach. *BMC Medical Education*, 22: 245.

8

Trauma-informed care

Principles, practices and benefits

Hannah Bailey

Case study

Richard's story

Before I had help, when I didn't know what to do, I would some-times go out in public in a very upset state. I was often taken to the emergency department by police and was left feeling misunder-stood and helpless. I didn't know what I wanted but I knew I didn't want to be handcuffed and taken in a police car.

A few months ago, I was handcuffed and taken to the hospi-tal where the staff were stern with me. The hospital was chaotic, bright, loud, and my anxiety increased. I couldn't speak and felt overwhelmed. I wanted to go home but couldn't get my words out and what I did say sounded angry. I said I hadn't done anything wrong, but it felt like no one believed me. I found myself shouting that no one was listening to me.

The nurse asking the questions was obviously frustrated with me. I heard her say to a colleague as she was leaving the room, that I was being difficult. I was left with a security guard, and I didn't know what was likely to happen next. I left the emergency depart-ment the first chance I had, feeling embarrassed and more scared than I had before going there.

It happened again a few months later and I was taken back to hospital by the police. A nurse met me when we arrived who spoke to me calmly and took her time, acknowledging I hadn't wanted to

DOI: 10.4324/9781003635604-8

come to the hospital. She asked if I had had a bad experience in the past and while I couldn't tell her, I could nod. She said that I was safe with her and that she would be looking after me for the rest of her shift. She explained what was going to happen, if I was willing to stay for an assessment with liaison services - something I'd never stayed long enough for before. She asked if I would like to go to quiet room with her to talk about the information needed to complete the referral. I agreed.

I was taken to a room with chairs where the lighting was a bit dimmer. There was information about trauma on the side and I was asked if I wanted a drink. It was peaceful in this room compared to the main area in the emergency department and the nurse took time to listen to me without any judgment about how I came to be here. She gave me some ideas of things to do to manage my anxiety while I was waiting for my assessment. Asking whether I had ever received any information about community services that were available, she pointed out some of the leaflets in the room, saying that I could have a look while I was waiting and take any that might be of interest. It was nice to have a choice about what I might want to do after I left the hospital. She said that she would be leaving me in the side room and that if I needed anything I could ring the bell. She also said she would pop in from time to time, to check that I was still okay, while I waited for the liaison team.

I felt a lot calmer, and it seemed as though people were listening. Previously, I had felt like a criminal even though the hospital was the last place I wanted to be. This time though, I was left feeling hopeful about being helped again in the future, if I needed it.

Introduction

Trauma-informed care (TIC) recognises that people face challenges, but they themselves are not the problem or problematic (NHS, 2025). When practising in a trauma-informed way, we understand that the way people act and speak, may be due to previous traumas, both within and outside of healthcare. Therefore, working with people in a way that upholds their dignity, ensuring the best possible mental and physical health outcomes, is fundamental to having a trauma-informed approach. We work collaboratively to understand how trauma may have had a lasting impact on someone's development and coping strategies, as well as their current reactions to situations which may be experienced as challenging (Elliott et al., 2005).

Chapter aims

This chapter focuses on providing a detailed understanding of trauma-informed approaches and includes information that aims to:

- Define and introducing the concept of trauma-informed care (TIC).
- Explore how TIC is beneficial to patients, carers and healthcare staff.
- Consider some simple changes that practitioners can make to begin working in a trauma-informed way.

Contemporary theory and practice

TIC is increasingly discussed as a way of improving patient experiences and outcomes, in the context of estimates that 70% of people will experience traumatic events in their lifetime (Kessler et al., 2017). Rather than being a specific intervention or treatment for trauma, TIC is an approach to working within clinical practice and organising clinical care in ways which recognise that many people using health and care services will have experienced trauma. This includes members of the healthcare team (National Trauma Transformation Programme, 2023) as explored in Chapter 9. The overall goal of TIC is to enable people who may find it challenging to access healthcare due to trauma to receive appropriate treatment (Office for Health Improvement and Disparities, 2022).

The UK government released its working definition of TIC in 2022 (Office for Health Improvement and Disparities, 2022), which aligns with the internationally recognised definition created by the United States Substance Abuse and Mental Health Services Administration (SAMHSA) (Substance Abuse and Mental Health Services Administration, 2014). This definition outlines some of the goals of TIC and includes the following statements of relevance to health and care practitioners:

1. TIC requires recognition that trauma effects groups and communities of people, as well as individuals, and that this trauma will impact on all areas of a person's functioning and development.
2. TIC aims to increase practitioners' understanding and awareness of how trauma impacts on someone's ability to access help and build close therapeutic relationships. Practitioners working in a trauma-informed way work collaboratively to empower people to make decisions about their care.
3. Lastly, TIC aims to stop re-traumatisation by healthcare services.

Key principles of TIC

There are six key principles of TIC used by the NHS (NHS, 2025; Office for Health Improvement and Disparities, 2022). These are safety, trust, choice, collaboration, empowerment and cultural considerations. The following statements explore what is meant by each of these principles.

Safety

Safety in the healthcare environment means protecting people from both physical and emotional harm (NHS, 2025; Office for Health Improvement and Disparities, 2022). It is important that people feel safe to ask for what they need and that organisations work to prevent re-traumatisation and ensure appropriate safeguarding (The National Association for People Abused in Childhood (NAPAC), 2024). SAMHSA (2014) highlights the need for safety to be defined by the individual receiving services or by the staff members working within a trauma-informed organisation.

Trustworthiness

This principle emphasises the need for organisations to build and maintain trust with staff, patients and the wider community (NHS, 2025; Office for Health Improvement and Disparities, 2022). According to NAPAC (2024), health organisations can achieve this by clearly outlining their policies and avoiding overpromising and underdelivering. Transparency in all decision-making processes is essential for trust (Substance Abuse and Mental Health Services Administration, 2014).

Choice

Choices about care need to be in the hands of the patient or service user (Kimberg, 2016), with the support of choice recognised as being central to empowerment (NHS, 2025; Office for Health Improvement and Disparities, 2022). Returning choice about care to the patient involves actively involving staff and patients in organisation-level decision-making, listening to their needs and acknowledging that it can be difficult to build trust after traumatic experiences (NAPAC, 2024).

Collaboration

Collaboration involves all levels of the organisation working with patients, carers and all members of the care team, regardless of status or job role, from cleaners to consultants (NHS, 2025; Office for Health Improvement and Disparities, 2022; Substance Abuse and Mental Health Services Administration, 2014). On an individual level, collaboration means recognising the unique knowledge and experience that patients and service users bring with them and then adopting that knowledge to work together towards a plan of care (Elliott et al., 2005). Collaborating helps reduce the risk of re-traumatisation as health professionals do not take a position of power over their patients and instead meet and work with them as equals (Elliott et al., 2005).

Empowerment

Sharing power at all levels of decision making within an organisation is fundamental to empowering people and communities (NAPAC, 2024; Substance Abuse and Mental Health Services Administration, 2014). NAPAC (2024) highlight that this includes validating concerns of staff, as well as their patients, listening to what they want and need and supporting them to make decisions and take action.

TIC recognises how experiencing trauma will potentially influence a person's coping strategies (Elliott et al., 2005). Helping people to see symptoms of depression, substance use or other traumatic responses, as an adaption and a way of managing a traumatic experience, can help people see themselves in a more positive light (Kimberg, 2016). This helps reduce feelings of low self-worth (NAPAC, 2024) and enables professionals to recognise the strengths and resilience of others (Kimberg, 2016).

Cultural, historical and gender considerations

The final key principle acknowledges and respects diversity and the challenges that whole communities can face (NHS, 2025; Office for Health Improvement and Disparities, 2022). There are several factors that can impact on someone's likelihood of experiencing trauma, including, but not limited to, gender, sexual orientation, disability, geographic factors and socioeconomic status.

Agboola et al. (2021) highlighted that race can contribute to the perception of agitation and aggression, suggesting that there is a need to consider our biases and how these impact on treatments offered. TIC would encourage reducing use of restraint, focusing instead on respecting personal space, setting limits, being clear about what the person wants and needs, and being mindful about our use of vocabulary and body language (Agboola et al., 2021). It is also important to be aware that culturally appropriate hand and arm gestures may be misinterpreted as expressions of agitation or aggression, by people who are unfamiliar with those cultures. Therefore, using a measurable or clinical description of specific actions which are observed, can reduce stigma (Agboola et al., 2021).

Table 8.1 uses Richard's case to provide a step-by-step example of how TIC can support a change in response to expressions of aggression and distress, and how this leads to different outcomes for staff, as well as for patients and service users.

Benefits of TIC

Implementing TIC in healthcare environments brings benefits for service users, carers and staff working in that environment. Nonetheless, there is currently limited research providing empirical evidence of the benefits of this approach, so further studies are required to assess the full impact of TIC across different areas of healthcare (Lewis et al., 2023). Other models

Table 8.1 An example of how TIC can change our response to perceived aggression

Non-trauma-informed approach	Trauma-informed approach
Richard is brought into the emergency department, appearing aggressive. The staff assume he's *'just another unruly individual'*.	Richard is brought into the emergency department, appearing aggressive. The staff recognise the potential signs of trauma and mental health crisis.
Staff respond to what is in front of them and do not make any attempt to understand what has happened to Richard for him to be acting in this way.	Staff respond in a trauma-informed way to attempt to support and de-escalate the situation.
1. Restraint: The staff restrain Richard without any attempt to understand his behaviour. They use physical force to subdue him and place him in a secluded room.	1. Create a safe environment: The staff remove Richard's handcuffs and offer him a comfortable, quiet space away from the main area to help him feel safe and reduce sensory overload.
2. Authoritative commands: Staff members shout commands at Richard, demanding him to *'calm down'* and *'stop shouting'*, further escalating his anxiety.	2. Respectful communication: Staff members approach Richard calmly and respectfully. They introduce themselves and explain their roles.
3. Judgemental attitude: The staff openly express their frustration, making derogatory comments about Richard's condition and behaviour, reinforcing his sense of shame and confusion.	3. Understanding: The staff acknowledge Richard's distress and validate his feelings, saying things like: *'It looks like you're going through a really tough time right now. We're here to help you'*.
4. Lack of communication: There is no attempt to explain the situation to Richard or to ask about his feelings or needs.	4. Collaboration: Richard is involved in his care, asking for his input and preferences. Staff provide clear explanations of the steps they are taking and seek his consent whenever possible.
Outcome: Richard feels even more frightened, isolated and misunderstood. His behaviour may escalate, and he may be less likely to seek help in the future.	5. Immediate needs: The staff assess Richard's immediate needs, such as hydration, warmth and any medical attention. They offer support and reassurance throughout the process.
	Outcome: Richard feels heard, respected and supported. His anxiety begins to decrease as he realises he is in a safe environment. This positive interaction may encourage him to seek help if experiencing a mental health crisis in the future.

of trauma-informed practice may identify other principles or pillars of such approaches, compared to those discussed here. Such principles may differ from researcher to researcher, highlighting the challenge of consistently operationalising TIC for the purpose of research and evaluation (Elliott et al., 2005; Sweeney et al., 2018).

Service users

The goals of TIC include patients and services users experiencing improved outcomes in their mental and physical health as well as re-traumatisation being avoided (Office for Health Improvement and Disparities, 2022). The use of collaboration and choice, alongside shared decision making, has been found to improve relationships between patients and staff and reduce patient anxiety (Goldstein et al., 2024). This can help with the subsequent disclosure of traumatic experiences.

People receiving TIC are more likely to be screened for symptoms relating to trauma, leading to better signposting to more appropriate interventions to support treatment for trauma symptoms (Berliner and Kolko, 2016). However, the principles of TIC need to be applied across the board, regardless of whether screening has taken place. Screening for the physical and psychological impacts of trauma may be more helpful in planning care, than screening for specific traumatic events (Kokokyi et al., 2021). Kokokyi et al. (2021) also state that when clinicians recognise the impact of racial and gender disparities, there is a better chance of health inequalities reducing.

Beyond screening for the mental health impacts of trauma, another potential benefit is that healthcare teams are able to provide information to patients about potential physiological effects of trauma, with the goal of improving long-term health outcomes (Grossman et al., 2021).

Carers

Examples of studies demonstrating the benefits of TIC for carers include studies where the parents of hospitalised children reported a positive response where staff had completed training in TIC (Simons et al., 2024). Simons et al. (2024) also found that parents reported it was helpful to have trauma screening for both the parent and the child, as this ultimately helped them access the treatment they needed. They also found that parents said that they would have been less likely to have realised the significance of the trauma, without this screening. Parents were also found to be more satisfied and confident in the care being provided, while children experienced fewer symptoms following discharge, when a trauma-informed approach had been used during hospital admission (Goldstein et al., 2024).

Staff members

Trauma-informed organisations recognise that staff can be affected by trauma in the same way their patients have been. Working in a trauma-informed organisation means that workloads, safety and the basic needs of staff are met (National Trauma Transformation Programme, 2023). There should be measures in place to prevent staff experiencing trauma associated with their work and the same principles of TIC apply to the staff experience (Kimberg, 2016; National Trauma Transformation Programme, 2023; Substance Abuse and Mental Health Services Administration, 2023). These include proactive measures, such as having role clarity and a job description, and reactive measures, for example in cases where a traumatic event occurs at work (National Trauma Transformation Programme, 2023). Staff should have the opportunity to learn to care for themselves, in their own unique way (Substance Abuse and Mental Health Services Administration, 2023), to reduce vicarious traumatisation in both the short and long term (Kimberg, 2016). Goldstein et al. (2024) found that staff had lower levels of burnout and that staff turnover reduced in organisations working in this way. Elisseou (2023) highlighted that burnout is a problem of the institution rather than the individual clinician and that some processes and systems of practice may increase the risk of burnout. Elisseou (2023) gave the example of feeling powerless when faced with a busy waiting room whilst being understaffed, and the likelihood that pressured team members will respond to this in the light of previous experiences where powerlessness has been experienced. Staff involved in the roll-out of TIC in one organisation reported feeling a sense of hope and optimism that they would be able to make a real difference to people's lives and health outcomes going forward (Champine et al., 2022).

Practitioners also experience the benefits which accrue for patients and service users where improved therapeutic relationships and feelings of empathy and support improved understanding of individuals' distress (Champine et al., 2022; Goldstein et al., 2024).

Implementation of TIC

TIC needs to be supported at both organisational and individual levels. Several frameworks have been developed to support TIC in different geographical locations (Children and Families Directorate, 2021; Public Health Wales NHS Trust, 2022; Substance Abuse and Mental Health Services Administration, 2014). Kimberg (2016) captures the themes of TIC and highlights that its foundation includes close working partnerships, support for health care professionals, ongoing monitoring and evaluation and trauma-informed values. All staff members need to be trained to understand trauma and its effects on individuals and colleagues, and how identity shapes the likelihood of encountering traumatic events. This training should also address the significance of historical and structural traumas (Kimberg, 2016).

There are three areas to build and develop around this foundation in a trauma-informed organisation. These are identified in Table 8.2 as the environment, screening for trauma and symptoms, and a planned response for disclosure.

Sweeney et al. (2018) highlighted that implementing a trauma-informed approach and working in this way can often feel challenging, as its implementation can lack clarity due to TIC not being a 'to-do' list that can be checked off as each task is completed. This view is shared by SAMHSA (2014).

Barriers to and enablers of TIC

There are challenges with the roll-out and study of TIC, and further research is required to support organisations to apply these principles (Stillerman et al., 2023). The lack of clear guidance, lack of definition (NHS, 2025), structure and evidence to support roll-out (Emsley et al., 2022), makes it challenging to measure effectiveness.

Funding arrangements and wider organisational as well as national support and guidance can improve or detract from the roll-out of these services (Huo et al., 2023; Sweeney et al., 2018). Emsley et al. (2022) found that there was a belief that without direct government support, TIC would not become embedded within England, and that Wales and Scotland had a more structured roll-out, supported by government services. Within organisations, high levels of engagement from staff and management alongside a willingness to change and work on organisational culture facilitate the

Table 8.2 Three areas to build and develop in a TIC organisation

The environment	This needs to be calm, safe and empowering to both patients and staff (Elliott et al., 2005). Environmental changes can include leaflets about trauma being available in public and private areas, ensuring cleanliness, and reduction in the brightness of lights and volume of noise (Kimberg, 2016; Kimberg and Wheeler, 2019). This is a care environment where staff strive to support patients to take as much control and ownership of their care and decision making as possible (Sweeney et al., 2018). Staff and patients are both more likely to report an increase in perceived safety when working in a trauma-informed environment (Lewis et al., 2023).
Screening for trauma and symptoms	Screening by staff for PTSD, depression, substance use and any trauma someone may have experienced, is routinely conducted (Kimberg, 2016). As part of this screening process, information about trauma and its effects is shared. This approach provides a safe way to introduce the topic of trauma to individuals who may feel uncomfortable discussing it with professionals. Screening can lead to a solution-focused approach to healthcare, rather than a problem-based approach (Sweeney et al., 2018). Thus, understanding what has happened to a person, what led to them being in front of you and what they need right now are more important than simply identifying what is 'wrong' with them in medical terms (The Office for Health Improvement and Disparities, 2022).
A planned response for disclosure.	The response of services when people disclose trauma needs to be planned in advance. This response may be a referral to a trauma-specific treatment programme, ongoing care onsite if working in a specialist area, or referral to local mental health services (Kimberg, 2016).

roll-out of TIC (Huo et al., 2023), while a lack of support from leadership is a barrier to implementation (Emsley et al., 2022).

Building new strategies into current procedures was found to be essential to sustaining TIC (Huo et al., 2023). For example, this may include a debrief for staff at every complex case discussion or introducing screening as part of the standard assessment process.

It can feel uncomfortable asking about trauma, so avoidance of asking can be a significant barrier to implementation, even when screening has become part of organisational policy (Berliner and Kolko, 2016). Equipping staff through training is therefore essential. All new employees who join an organisation should have TIC training when they begin as part of their induction (Huo et al.,

2023) to ensure that from the start of their career they are able to provide and understand this way of working. Training in TIC means that staff are more confident in understanding the consequences of trauma and the impacts of broader inequalities experienced by service users (Kokokyi et al., 2021).

Similarly, long-standing staff at all levels of an organisation require regular ongoing training (Huo et al., 2023). An inability of services to prioritise training and support staff to attend has been found as a barrier to rolling out TIC (Huo et al., 2023). Similarly, training in TIC must be treated as a core clinical intervention, rather than something someone completes only if they have a special interest in trauma (Okoli et al., 2024). In research looking at the sustainability of initial roll-outs, it was found that over 3 years, levels of staff training could remain consistent if supported by organisations after the initial roll-out (Snider et al., 2023).

In organisations where TIC was rolled out in ways that involved interagency working and potentially training of external agencies, this supported delivery of TIC (Huo et al., 2023; Simons et al., 2024). Where agencies outside of the direct healthcare environment did not work in a trauma-informed way this can undo some of the work completed within settings that have adopted TIC, leading to a reduction in trust (Huo et al., 2023). An analysis by Bulford et al. (2024) highlighted partnership working and effective communication between services as facilitators of TIC.

Themes often seen in all aspects of healthcare change and transformation, and which present barriers to the roll-out and implementation of TIC, are lack of time, lack of flexibility in working practices and a lack of collaborative working between teams (Bulford et al., 2024; Huo et al., 2023; Simons et al., 2024).

Tools for now: small changes that can make a big difference

We, as individual healthcare practitioners, can deliver trauma-informed support and work in ways that improve the experience of patients and service users.

Enquiring about trauma

One way we can support individuals is by shifting our own perspective from asking, *'What is wrong with this person?'* to considering, *'What has happened to this person?'* (Greenwald et al., 2023). When working in a trauma-informed way, we assume that all people may have experienced trauma, as well as asking about potentially traumatic experiences. In this way, we can effectively signpost each person and provide information on the potential impact of trauma on physical health.

We need to be prepared to ask patients and service users about their experiences of trauma and for this to be a normal and routine part of screening and assessment (Sweeney et al., 2018). We might ask whether someone has experienced anything that could make it hard to see a healthcare professional, or explicitly ask if they have experienced trauma relating to receiving healthcare (Greenwald et al., 2023).

Some people may choose not to disclose, and it is important to note that people do not have to answer if they do not want to. If someone does share experiences of trauma or abuse, it is recommended that we respond in the following ways (Sweeney et al., 2018):

- Provide reassurance and encouragement that disclosure is helpful and a positive thing.
- Do not ask for specific details about the trauma they may have experienced.
- Ask about their experiences of telling people in the past. Have people been helpful? If so, what was helpful?
- Offer support around trauma and complete a referral to trauma services if required.
- Check that the person is currently safe.
- And check their emotional state at the end of the appointment.

Longer-term changes: rolling out a trauma-informed approach

The roll-out of TIC needs support at all levels of an organisation and is likely to require active assessment and involvement from teams and individuals who are passionate about this work (SAMHSA, 2023).

If you want to learn more about the roll-out of TIC, whether at a departmental, ward or organisational level, SAMHSA (2023) has created an implementation guide to help support this. The first step towards a trauma-informed organisation is undertaking a baseline assessment so that any successes and challenges that follow can be identified, measured and recorded.

This assessment is for all staff in an organisation and requires openness and honesty about their experiences. An example of a self-assessment tool can be found online at the Trauma Informed Care Project (n.d. – see reference list).

Following the assessment, a plan can be created around the areas to work on for implementation, using the 10 implementation domains (SAMHSA, 2023):

1. Governance and leadership
2. Training and workforce development
3. Cross-sector collaboration
4. Financing
5. Physical environment
6. Engagement and involvement
7. Screening, assessment and treatment services
8. Progress monitoring and quality assurance
9. Policy
10. Evaluation

Each of these domains is required for providing TIC and several aspects of development may be covered in each. For example, training and workforce development includes training needs of teams as well as in developing person-centred plans for responding to, and being supported with, managing challenging and potentially trauma-inducing, situations.

Following the implementation of the plan and work on the 10 areas, evaluation of the TIC changes takes place, and policies will need to be adapted to ensure that TIC continues to be followed at the end of the initial implementation stage.

Summary of learning points

This chapter has explored TIC and its impact on teams and patients within the healthcare environment:

- TIC continues to be a challenging area to research or fully evaluate due to the existence of a range of definitions and implementation strategies.
- There are benefits of TIC for patients, carers and healthcare staff, alongside positive consequences for the wider organisation.

- TIC requires education, training, information and collaboration at all levels of an organisation.
- There are tools we can use as individuals to provide TIC, even if our organisation has not yet fully implemented this approach into our workplace.

Questions for reflection and discussion

1. In the organisation where you work, how are the principles of TIC applied to staff as well as to patients and service users? How is TIC applied within your team?
2. In your area of practice, how might the topic of trauma be introduced to patients and carers, whether adults or children?
3. Consider the spaces used by patients and carers in your workplace. How can a trauma-informed approach be promoted in these environments? For example, is literature available for people to pick up in both public and private areas? Is the space calm and does it convey a sense of compassion, or is it purely functional or clinical?
4. Have patients and carers been asked about their experience of the environment in which your services are provided? How could collaboration support environmental changes alongside a growing understanding of what it feels like to receive services?
5. Think about the communities you work with. How are they uniquely impacted by trauma? Consider individuals, family units and the wider community as well as the impact of, for example, race, gender, socio-economic standing, geographical challenges and historical events.

Recommended follow-up reading

Evans, A. and Coccoma, P. (2017). *Trauma-informed care: How neuroscience influences practice* (Explorations in mental health). Abingdon: Routledge.

Gerber, M.R. (2019). *Trauma-informed healthcare approaches: A guide for primary care*. Boston: Springer.

Melillo, A., Sansone, N., Allan, J., Gill, N., Herrman, H., Cano, G.M., Rodrigues, M., Savage, M. and Galderisi, S. (2025). Recovery-oriented and trauma-informed care for people with mental disorders to promote human rights and quality of mental health care: A scoping review. *BMC Psychiatry*, 25(1): 1–22.

Reeves, E. (2015). A synthesis of the literature on trauma-informed care. *Issues in Mental Health Nursing*, 36(9): 698–709.

Treisman, K. (2024). *Trauma-informed health care: A reflective guide for improving care and services*. London: Jessica Kingsley Publishers.

References

Agboola, I.K., Coupet, E. and Wong, A.H. (2021). The coats that we can take off and the ones we can't": The role of. *Annals of Emergency Medicine*, 77(5): 493–498.

Berliner, L. and Kolko, D.J. (2016). Trauma informed care: A commentary and critique. *Child Maltreatment*, 21(2): 168–172.

Bulford, E., Baloch, S., Neil, J. and Hegarty, K. (2024). Primary healthcare practitioners' perspectives on trauma-informed primary care: A systematic review. *BMC Primary Care*, 25: 336.

Champine, R.B., Hoffman, E.E., Matlin, S.L., Strambler, M.J. and Tebes, J.K. (2022). "What does it mean to be trauma-informed?": A mixed-methods study of a trauma-informed community initiative. *Journal of Child and Family Studies*. 31: 459–472.

Children and Families Directorate (2021). *Trauma-informed practice: A toolkit for Scotland*. Scottish Government. https://www.gov.scot/publications/trauma-informed-practice-toolkit-scotland/documents/[Accessed 16th June 2025].

Elisseou, S. (2023). Trauma-informed care: A missing link in addressing burnout. *Journal of Healthcare Leadership*, 15: 169–173.

Elliott, D.E., Fallot, R.D., Markoff, L. and Reed, B.G. (2005). Trauma-informed or trauma-denied: Principles and implementation of trauma-informed services for women. *Journal of Community Psychology*, 33(4): 461–477.

Emsley, E., Smith, J., Martin, D. and Lewis, N.V. (2022). Trauma-informed care in the UK: Where are we? A qualitative study of health policies and professional perspectives. *BMC Health Services Research*, 22: 1164.

Goldstein, E., Chokshi, B., Melendez-Torres, G.J., Rios, A., Jelley, M. and Lewis-O'Connor, A. (2024). Effectiveness of trauma-informed care implementation in health care settings: Systematic review of reviews and realist synthesis. *The Permanente Journal*, 28(1): 135–150.

Greenwald, A., Kelly, A., Mathew, T. and Thomas, L. (2023). Trauma-informed care in the emergency department: Concepts and recommendations for integrating practices into emergency medicine. *Medical Education Online*, 28(1): 1–8.

Grossman, S., Cooper, Z., Buxton, H., Hendrickson, S., Lewis-O'Connor, A., Stevens, J., Wong, L.-Y. and Bonne, S. (2021). Trauma-informed care: Recognizing and resisting re-traumatization in healthcare. *Trauma Surgery and Acute Care Open*, 6(1): e000815.

Huo, Y., Couzner, L., Windsor, T., Laver, T., Dissanayaka, N.N. and Cations, N. (2023). Barriers and enablers for the implementation of trauma-informed care in healthcare settings: A systematic review. *Implementation Science Communications*, 4: 49.

Kessler, R.C., Aguilar-Gaxiola, S., Alonso, J., Benjet, C., Bromet, E.J., Cardoso, G., Degenhardt, L., de Girolamo, G., Dinolova, R.V., Ferry, F. and Florescu, S. (2017). Trauma and PTSD in the WHO World Mental Health Surveys. *European Journal of Psychotraumatology*, 8(5): p1353383.

Kimberg, L.S. (2016). Trauma and trauma-informed care. In: King, T.E., Wheeler, M.B., Bindman, A.B., Fernandez, A., Grumbach, K., Schillinger, D. and Villela, T.J (eds) *Medical management of vulnerable and underserved patients: Principles, practice, and populations* (2nd ed.). New York: McGraw Hill.

Kimberg, L.S. and Wheeler, M. (2019). Trauma and trauma-informed care. In: Gerber, M.R. (ed) *Trauma-informed healthcare approaches: A guide for primary care*. Boston: Springer.

Kokokyi, S., Klest, B. and Anstey, H. (2021). A patient-oriented research approach to assessing patients' and primary care physicians' opinions on trauma-informed care. *PLOS One*, 16(7): e0254266.

Lewis, N.V., Bierce, A., Feder, G.S., Macleod, J., Turner, K.M., Zammit, S. and Dawson, S. (2023). Trauma-informed approached in primary healthcare and community mental healthcare: A mixed methods systematic review of organisational change interventions. *Health and social care in the community*, 2023: 4475114.

NAPAC (National Association for People Abused in Childhood). (2024). *What are the six key principles of a trauma-informed approach?* https://napac.org.uk/blog-what-are-the-six-key-principles-of-a-trauma-informed-approach/ [Accessed 10th February 2025].

National Trauma Transformation Programme. (2023). *A roadmap for creating trauma-informed and responsive change: Guidance for organisations, systems and workforces in Scotland*. https://www.traumatransformation.scot/implementation/ [Accessed 6th February 2025].

NHS. (2025). *Trauma informed practice*. https://safeguarding-guide.nhs.uk/context-of-NHS-safeguarding/s2-03/ [Accessed 5th February 2025].

Office for Health Improvement and Disparities. (2022). *Working definition of trauma-informed practice*. https://www.gov.uk/government/publications/working-definition-of-trauma-informed-practice/working-definition-of-trauma-informed-practice [Accessed 5th February 2025].

Okoli, D., Dobson, M., Schneiderhan, J., Moravek, M., Stojan, J. and Haas, M. (2024). 12 tips for implementing trauma-informed care within undergraduate medical education. *MedEdPublish*, 14: 281.

Public Health Wales NHS Trust. (2022). *Trauma-informed Wales: A societal approach to understanding, preventing and supporting the impacts of trauma and adversity*. https://traumaframeworkcymru.com/wp-content/uploads/2022/07/Trauma-Informed-Wales-Framework.pdf [Accessed 4th March 2025].

Simons, M., Harvey, G., McMillan, L., Ryan, E.G., De Young, A.G., McPhail, S.M., Kularatna, S., Senanayake, S., Kimble, R. and Tyack, Z. (2024). Implementation outcomes of a digital, trauma-informed care, educational intervention targeting health professionals in a paediatric burns setting: A mixed methods process evaluation. *Burns*, 50(6): 1690–1703.

Snider, M.D.H., Taylor, R.M., Bills, L.J., Hutchinson, S.L., Steinman, S.A. and Herschell, A.D. (2023). Implementing trauma-informed care through a learning collaborative: A theory-driven analysis of sustainability. *Community Mental Health Journal*, 59: 881–893.

Stillerman, A., Altman, L., Peña, G., Cua, G., Goben, A., Walden, A.L. and Atkins, M.S. (2023). Advancing trauma-informed care in hospitals: The time is now. *The Permanente Journal*, 27(1): 16–19.

Substance Abuse and Mental Health Services Administration (SAMHSA). (2014). *SAMHSA's concept or trauma and guidance for a trauma-informed approach*. Rockville: U.S. Department of Health and Human Services.

Substance Abuse and Mental Health Services Administration (SAMHSA). (2023) *Practical guide for implementing a trauma-informed approach*. Rockville: National Mental Health and Substance Use Policy Laboratory.

Sweeney, A., Filson, B., Kennedy, A., Collinson, L. and Gillard, S. (2018). A paradigm shift: Relationships in trauma-informed mental health services. *BJPsych Advances*, 24(5): 319–333.

Trauma-Informed Care Project. (n.d.). *Guide to completing the agency self-assessment*. http://www.traumainformedcareproject.org/resources/Trauam%20 Informed%20Organizational%20Survey_9_13.pdf [Accessed 4th March 2025].

9

The traumatised practitioner

Self-awareness, supervision and reflective practice

Sarah Housden

Case study

Alison's story

Part of my role is to carry out assessments with people who are at risk due to their mental health before they are referred into secondary services. On the whole, since overcoming the anxiety of being newly qualified and making it through those first 12 months, I have not struggled to keep my personal and professional lives separate. There were though, two occasions, where I was profoundly affected by other people's experiences. In the first situation, I anticipated my reaction, while in the second, I was caught by surprise.

The first scenario involved assessing a lady who had undergone termination of pregnancy for medical reasons due to advice from doctors because of a cancer diagnosis for which she was awaiting treatment. However, she had found out after the termination that it could have been safe to continue with the pregnancy. Understandably, this devastated her. This was further complicated by her reaching the top of the waiting list for her hysterectomy two weeks after the termination. All this had taken place a few weeks before she met with me due to experiencing suicidal thoughts, partly in reaction to the knowledge that she would not be able to try again to have her much-wanted baby. Having experienced miscarriages

DOI: 10.4324/9781003635604-9

myself and having a medical condition that led to my own hyster-ectomy, I felt this woman's pain on a deep level. I went to the office of a female colleague and asked her for the space to cry about how awful the things this patient had experienced were. I wanted to get it all out of my system before going to see her face to face. Having this space to talk through my understanding of the patient's expe-riences, alongside my experiences and my feelings, I was able to maintain professionalism during the assessment, and afterwards, I requested time for a more formal supervision where I was able to express the emotions held in throughout that assessment.

The second situation involved assessing a man who appeared to meet the criteria for a neurodiversity diagnosis and who had recently been through a messy relationship break-up. It seemed that he did not realise the extent of the abuse within the rela-tionship, which included relentless bullying around his reaction to losing his parents. His situation touched me because of my own neurodiversity diagnosis combined with the recent death of a close family member. During the assessment, in validating his experiences of grief and loss that had been previously invalidated and victimised, I found myself unable to hold back my tears. In fact, we cried together. I apologised for this, although he said he found it comforting and highly validating of his experiences. After the assessment, I went straight to my manager's office and sat crying for ten minutes before I was able to say what had made me so upset. In this scenario, the blurring of my own emotions impacted my confidence in my ability to judge risk and we there-fore arranged a further review for this patient with an advanced nurse practitioner within our team.

Introduction

This chapter explores how health and social care practitioners can work in ways which help keep us emotionally and psychologically safe, recognis-ing that we and our colleagues may have experienced adverse childhood events, as well as trauma at any stage of life. Furthermore, health and care practitioners are likely to work with patients and service users with diverse histories, which could include traumatic events. Therefore, as well as potentially experiencing our own traumas throughout life, with which we may or may not have come to terms, we are also at risk of experiencing secondary traumatic stress (STS) or vicarious trauma (VT) due to being exposed to the traumas of our patients and service users (Al Barmawi et al., 2025; Jimenez et al., 2021).

Traditional models of supervision within health settings are unlikely to meet the needs of healthcare practitioners affected in these ways. Instead, awareness of and skill in providing supportive, reflective and trauma-informed supervision (McGarva et al., 2024) are essential for all those with responsibilities for supervising and supporting frontline health and care practitioners.

Chapter aims

This chapter considers elements of trauma-informed practice from the perspective of the healthcare practitioner, including exploration of:

- Self-awareness and the ability to explore personal triggers and reactions in a professional way.
- Using reflective supervision effectively to promote and maintain wellbeing in the workplace and beyond.
- The limits of clinical supervision, including situations that might reduce openness, honesty and trust within the supervisory relationship.
- Supporting colleagues with experience of trauma.
- Ways to promote our own wellbeing as practitioners together with considerations around the responsibilities of the wider organisation.

Contemporary theory and practice

Although under-researched, evidence suggests that healthcare workers have higher numbers of adverse childhood experiences (ACEs) than the general population (Bouchard and Rainbow, 2021; Clark and Aboueissa, 2021). Mercer et al. (2023) found that ACEs among health and social care workers were frequently reported and occurred more often than in the general population. They were also associated with several negative personal and professional outcomes, including poor physical and mental health, and workplace stress. Esaki and Larkin (2018) found that there was a high incidence of ACEs among children's service providers signalling a need for research demonstrating the potential impacts on compassion fatigue, secondary traumatic effects and vicarious trauma. Compassion fatigue is also a potential risk factor for care providers' mental health and has led to increased numbers leaving the nursing profession (Nolte et al., 2017).

Conti-O'Hare (2002) wrote about the nurse as a 'wounded healer', describing a prevalence of nurses who have their own psychological wounds and suggesting that healthcare workers must undertake their own healing journey in the process of caring for others. It is more important than ever for nurses and AHPs, as well as students, to practise self-awareness and develop understanding of their personal narratives and emotional triggers, particularly in a healthcare system that can be perceived as neglecting those working within it.

We can protect ourselves with regular supervision, peer support, diverse caseloads, specific trauma training and a culture, which validates vicarious trauma (Sutton et al., 2022). Clinicians with their own trauma history might also consider engaging in therapy and self-reflection, to better understand emotional triggers.

The nature of working in healthcare means that practitioners can be exposed to emotionally challenging and potentially traumatic situations through daily encounters with illness, injury, suffering and death (Dar et al., 2024). This can lead to psychological trauma, which may have considerable impact on the personal and professional lives of practitioners, and particularly on the ongoing development of student practitioners (Burr et al., 2025). Understanding the nature of trauma and implementing evidence-based support strategies are fundamental to reducing staff turnover and to maintaining a robust and resilient workforce across health and care settings.

Healthcare professionals are particularly susceptible to indirect forms of trauma due to the empathic nature of this work (Moudatsou et al., 2020). Vicarious trauma resulting from exposure to the traumatic stories and experiences of others can have a cumulative negative effect on the physical and mental health of team members (Dar et al., 2024). Secondary trauma (Al Barmawi et al., 2025) involves the development of PTSD-like symptoms without directly witnessing or being involved in a traumatic event. Thus, the traumatising event of a patient can become a traumatising event for the healthcare professional in ways which effect wellbeing. This can show itself in the form of compassion fatigue and professional burnout (Noor et al., 2025).

Moral injury and ethical dilemmas (Rabin et al., 2023) also occur on a regular basis in healthcare settings. An example of this is where a person witnesses actions which conflict with their moral or ethical beliefs and fail (or are unable) to prevent these events from happening, or worse still, find themselves engaging in and contributing to such events. In the context of contemporary healthcare, some of these dilemmas will be instigated by resource shortages and organisational pressures, which can limit opportunities to provide high-quality care (Kerasidou, 2019). Thus, an individual can find themselves having to make life and death decisions about patients, which can lead to escalating feelings of distress, guilt, shame and anger, contributing to long-term psychological, spiritual or social distress (Webb et al., 2024).

Such situations were seen during the COVID-19 pandemic, which placed additional burdens on already-stretched and under-resourced healthcare systems, organisations, leaders and workers (Morris et al., 2025). The increased workload, fear of infection, increasingly complex ethical dilemmas and exposure to widespread morbidity left many healthcare practitioners vulnerable to trauma (Williamson et al., 2023).

Self-awareness around trauma and personal triggers

Self-awareness enables healthcare workers to navigate complex situations and to maintain a professional approach as they traverse the internal landscape of emotions, values and motivations, alongside recognising the effects of external stressors (Younas et al., 2020). Self-awareness makes it more likely that we can avoid projecting our personal feelings and concerns onto others, leading to a better understanding of the needs of our patients and colleagues (Harley, 2024). By contrast, unrecognised and thus, unacknowledged emotions can present a barrier to working effectively with others and can potentially contribute to poor judgements and clinical errors.

The ability to see ourselves as we are, and to recognise our own strengths and limitations, contributes to being able to work in a person-centred way and to developing empathic and meaningful connections with colleagues, patients and their families, leading to improved communication and better relationships (Harley, 2024). Understanding our own feelings also gives us the capacity to better understand the feelings and experiences of others, thus supporting the delivery of more holistic and individualised care.

Individuals who recognise the need to take responsibility for their own wellbeing, including caring for their emotional and psychological health, are more likely to set boundaries, seek support and engage in activities that promote physical and mental health (Sist et al., 2022).

Ethical guidelines and professional standards in healthcare emphasise the importance of self-awareness and the management of personal wellbeing, especially in relation to managing personal experiences of trauma (HCPC, 2022; RCN, 2024). Self-awareness plays a key role in facilitating and promoting safety, trustworthiness, choice, collaboration and empowerment within health and care settings and relationships.

Reflective practice

Reflective practice involves deliberately thinking through emotions, past experiences, current circumstances and the many values, beliefs and potential biases that we bring to our roles in healthcare practice. This can involve using a structured approach (Esterhuizen, 2022) with prompts to explore a specific situation to identify factors including emotional responses, to promote understanding of why events occurred as they did. The overall aim is to consider alternative actions that could have been taken and plans for improving future action based on these insights.

Reflection can enhance self-awareness, refine clinical decision-making skills and facilitate more effective person-centred care (NMC, 2024). It supports continuous learning and development, playing a part in building emotional resilience, by equipping practitioners with improved coping mechanisms. It may also help individuals manage symptoms of vicarious trauma as the healthcare worker consciously separates themselves from their exposure to traumatic material, compartmentalising those experiences in a separate part of the conscious mind (Hazen et al., 2020).

Reflective supervision

Reflection involves intentionally slowing down and focusing attention on emotional responses, thereby helping the healthcare practitioner to recognise the significance of their feelings within the context of their professional interactions. For this, there needs to be sufficient time in an emotionally and psychologically safe space, which can be created through reflective supervision. Enablers of effective supervision identified by Rothwell et al. (2021) included regular supervision, occurring within protected time and in a private space, and delivered flexibly. Regularity ensures that supervision sessions occur consistently and predictably, providing a reliable space for healthcare practitioners to actively engage with in-depth thinking about their work.

Reflective supervision plays a key role in enhancing the quality of care provided by health and care workers, facilitating development of reflective practice skills as well as specific professional competencies. This enables healthcare practitioners to acquire more extensive knowledge as well as enhancing their overall competence across the domains of professional practice. This, in turn, equips us with insights to more effectively recognise and address the needs of patients and service users who have experienced trauma.

Furthermore, reflective supervision has a positive impact on the supervisory relationship itself. It can shift the dynamic away from a more traditional, directive approach towards a relationship that is characterised by greater collaboration and mutual respect. This can also encourage supervisees to take a more active role in their learning and to develop their own problem-solving abilities (Markey et al., 2020). In the context of providing trauma-informed services, a strong supervisory relationship built on trust and open communication is vital to providing effective guidance and support to the workforce.

Trauma-informed principles of safety, trustworthiness, collaboration, empowerment and cultural sensitivity each need to be integrated into the supervisory process. This ensures that supervisees are properly supported and feel understood. The intentional integration of trauma-informed principles at the supervisory level ensures that the approach taken to interacting with staff who are trauma survivors is sensitive, ethical and likely to promote recovery.

Of course, supervisors also need to develop a deeper understanding of their own inner landscape and emotional reactions. The idea of a supervisor who lacks self-awareness is highly problematic, but not unheard of, in health and care settings. Identifying personal triggers and potential biases that could influence interactions with supervisees is therefore essential to the ability of clinical supervisors to listen well and to make balanced decisions.

Emotionally intelligent supervisors are better equipped to navigate complex interpersonal dynamics within their teams, effectively managing any conflicts that arise and developing a positive work culture where everyone feels valued and understood (Prezerakos, 2018). The ability to remain calm and composed under pressure allows supervisors to make well-considered decisions, even in challenging and emotionally charged situations.

Openness, honesty and trust in healthcare supervision

Effective clinical supervision plays an important role in ensuring the quality of patient care and in fostering the professional development of healthcare professionals. This requires openness, honesty and the building of trust within the supervisory relationship. Openness involves unimpeded discussion around ideas and concerns between the supervisor and supervisee in an environment where individuals feel comfortable to express thoughts, feelings and perspectives without fear of negative repercussions (Mostafa et al., 2025). This includes acknowledging mistakes, openly discussing challenges and providing honest feedback. Establishing an environment in which any uncertainties, alongside emotional needs and potentially, the need for additional training can be expressed without feeling judged, is central to developing a supportive supervisory relationship. This enables healthcare professionals to seek support, admit their limits and engage in authentic and in-depth reflection, thus supporting self-awareness and professional development. Such an open culture creates an environment for learning from experience where challenges are seen as opportunities for growth rather than an occasion for blame or shame (Berger and Quiros, 2014; McGarva et al., 2024; Mostafa et al., 2025).

However, achieving open communication in healthcare supervision can be impeded by the complex interplay between individual, relational and organisational factors. Individual factors include personal characteristics, which can present a barrier to open discussions. Some individuals may struggle, for example, to express their thoughts and concerns, or to listen and respond positively to feedback. This can lead to an escalation of emotional and communication challenges, especially where sensitive topics around performance are being discussed (Rothwell et al., 2021).

Negative attitudes, whether towards patients, supervisors or other team members, can also create a hostile atmosphere that makes open conversations more difficult. Such attitudes might be seen in a lack of empathy or unwillingness to engage with in-depth supervisory discussions. Similarly, a lack of self-confidence can make a person hesitant to voice their opinions or openly discuss any struggles with their supervisors for fear of seeming incompetent. Such factors can lead to supervisee–supervisor interactions, which lack depth and honesty (Sellers et al., 2016).

The hierarchical nature of healthcare often creates a dynamic where supervisees may be apprehensive about being completely honest with their supervisors due to fear of negative consequences (Safavi and Bouzari, 2025). The inherent power differential means that supervisees might worry about receiving poor evaluations, facing disciplinary action or even losing their job if they are honest about their shortcomings. Such fears are not necessarily unjustified where the supervisor is not working in a trauma informed way.

The broader organisational context also influences the quality of communication within supervisory relationships. A lack of support from senior managers can undermine efforts to promote open communication. If the organisation does not prioritise or resource initiatives aimed at improving communication skills and developing a supportive supervisory culture, open dialogue is less likely to flourish. Heavy workloads and time constraints can be major barriers to effective communication and regular supervision. When healthcare professionals are burdened with excessive tasks and limited time, opportunities for in-depth supervisory interactions and meaningful discussions are reduced, again leading to more superficial conversations (Rothwell et al., 2021).

Team managers therefore occupy a pivotal position in the implementation and oversight of trauma support initiatives within health and care organisations. Part of being responsible for the implementation of policies and procedures aimed at promoting workforce wellbeing involves ensuring that all members of the workforce have access to the resources they need.

Supporting colleagues with experience of trauma

Adopting a trauma-informed approach within healthcare organisations represents a fundamental shift in how care is delivered and how staff are supported, because this approach moves away from asking *'What's wrong with you?'* to understanding *'What happened to you?'* It emphasises creating an environment that prioritises safety, trustworthiness, transparency, collaboration, empowerment, choice and cultural sensitivity, for patients and for the health and care workforce.

Integrating knowledge about trauma into all organisational policies, procedures and practices is essential, with a conscious effort needed to avoid re-traumatising others, including our colleagues, within the workplace. A trauma-informed approach creates a more supportive and understanding work environment for healthcare practitioners, which requires a commitment to developing a culture of wellbeing and safety. This requires ongoing training for all staff members, clinical and non-clinical, and a strategic approach to developing an organisation which embodies person-centred and trauma-informed approaches.

It can sometimes be the case that managers within a workplace see themselves as being exempt from the need for training in empathy, advanced communication skills, self-care and self-awareness. However, if trauma-informed practice is to be effective, then relevant training, policies and procedures need to be integrated into all job roles and into everyday practice. Only then will colleagues know that they have permission to take time out of the working day to support one another and to normalise reflection on their emotional reactions to traumatising work. Whether working in an emergency department, in a care home for older people or in a primary care administration role, all people involved in health and care work will at times come across situations, which challenge our emotional wellbeing. Being able to turn to colleagues to talk things through, as Alison does in the case study at the start of this chapter, is vital to workplace wellbeing. Recognising our personal triggers and the vicarious, secondary and moral traumas occurring in the workplace are key to the ability of healthcare practitioners, teams and organisations, moving beyond surviving, to thriving. The development of self-nurturing skills and the ability to support colleagues in professional and trauma-informed ways is integral to trauma-informed practice. Developing these skills requires a reflective approach to practice.

All team members need to be aware of and able to recognise signs and symptoms of historic, vicarious, secondary and moral trauma, alongside burnout, in their colleagues. It is essential to be equipped with the skills to initiate supportive conversations and to guide individuals towards wider support mechanisms, such as occupational health services, workplace counselling, wellbeing teams or mental health services.

We all play a role in fostering a team environment where open communication and mutual support are encouraged, helping to create a safer workplace for staff members who may be struggling with the impact of any kind of traumatic experiences – whenever these occurred.

Ultimately, effective management is essential for translating an organisation's commitment to the wellbeing of its workforce, into tangible and readily accessible systems of support, which are effective at a team level (Vang, 2023). While challenges exist, the benefits of implementing such approaches are significant.

Tools for now: small changes that can make a big difference

Balancing work with the rest of life

Maintaining a healthy work–life balance is essential for the wellbeing of healthcare professionals, playing a central role in the prevention of compassion fatigue and burnout as well as reducing the long-term effects of vicarious, secondary and moral trauma. Working long shifts and the pattern of these can make it challenging to reserve time and energy for investing in hobbies, friends and families, and in rest. An imbalance in how we spend the limited hours in each week can lead to exacerbations in stress and fatigue, whilst reducing job satisfaction and our overall wellbeing.

Purposively achieving a healthier work–life balance involves effectively managing time and energy to meet both professional and personal commitments, as well as focusing on self-care. Healthcare organisations have a responsibility to prevent excessive workloads, offer flexible work arrangements where possible, signpost to mental health resources and establish reasonably predictable shift patterns. Aiming for homes and workplaces to be separate and for electronic devices to be switched off where possible so that periods of downtime from work-related messages are achievable, should be encouraged by managers. This includes supporting all members of the workforce to learn to say no to additional commitments, particularly when they are feeling overwhelmed.

Managing emotional reactions

The following practices can be helpful for managing our emotional reactions, supporting the development of self-awareness and enhancing emotional regulation.

1. Mindfulness practices, such as meditation and deep breathing exercises, can help us become more present and aware of our emotions without judgement, allowing us to make a more thoughtful response rather than giving an immediate reaction.
2. Self-regulation techniques, including recognising triggers and practising relaxation, are crucial for managing intense emotional responses. Grounding exercises can also be helpful in bringing focus to the present moment when feeling overwhelmed by emotional reactions (see the tools described in Chapter 4).
3. Growing our social connections, engaging in hobbies and seeking mental health support can contribute to overall emotional wellbeing.
4. Self-reflection through journalling can play a significant role in identifying triggers and managing emotional reactions. Regularly writing down thoughts and feelings can help reveal patterns and triggers that might not be immediately obvious.
5. Seeking feedback from colleagues, supervisors or mentors provides valuable external perspectives on how our emotional responses are perceived by others, which can enhance self-awareness and inform self-management strategies.

Self-care strategies for managing stress and trauma

Prioritising self-care is a fundamental aspect of supporting wellbeing and reducing the impact of stress and trauma. These include:

1. Ensuring adequate sleep by practising good sleep hygiene, such as maintaining a consistent sleep schedule and creating a restful sleep environment.
2. Prioritising healthy eating by maintaining a balanced diet and staying well-hydrated.
3. Regular physical exercise as part of managing stress.

Enhancing personal resilience

A call to greater resilience is sometimes used by healthcare managers in a way that focuses on the responsibility of individuals to protect their own wellbeing, whilst neglecting the role of the wider team and organisation in supporting everyone's wellbeing. This can lead to a situation where people who are traumatised are blamed for their reactions to accumulated stressors by being told that they lack resilience. Such an approach is destructive to the wellbeing of the individual and to the wider team, as well as to patients where a similar ethos of 'blaming the victim' is more widely adopted. This is the very opposite of trauma-informed care. Instead, resilience is best promoted in the context of groups of individuals working together. In that context, techniques for enhancing resilience can include:

1. Cultivating a positive mindset within the team by focusing on all that is being achieved, and learning from challenges, as well as practising gratitude.
2. Developing adaptive coping skills together, such as discussing ways to reframe the way a team is thinking about a situation or patient. This can help in managing stress and maintaining composure in high-pressure situations.
3. Establishing strong support systems by building connections between colleagues, with mentors and through professional networks, which may provide outlets for sharing experiences and seeking guidance.

Ideas for longer-term: developing trauma-informed workplaces

Those holding managerial roles within health and care organisations need to work to promote:

- Clear policies and protocols for trauma-informed reflective supervision being aligned with the development and implementation of guidance on best practice.
- Protected time and adequate resources being allocated for regular supervision sessions.
- Training for supervisors on the principles and practice of trauma-informed supervision, with specific attention to working with and reducing vicarious trauma.
- Ongoing professional development for supervisors in trauma-informed supervisory practice.

- An organisational culture that fosters open communication and mutual respect, alongside emotional and psychological safety within supervisory relationships and across all teams.
- Access to reflective supervision, peer support networks and mentorship opportunities for all supervisors, to address the risk of vicarious trauma and burnout.
- Recognition of the unique demands placed on supervisors in trauma-informed settings.

Critical incident stress management (CISM) and debriefing protocols

Critical incident stress management (CISM) offers a structured approach to addressing the impact of highly stressful critical incidents on individuals and teams. Critical incident stress debriefing (CISD) is a key component of CISM, involving a facilitator-led group process conducted soon after a traumatic event. The primary goals of CISD are to facilitate emotional processing of the event, normalising the range of reactions individuals may experience and providing guidance on stress management techniques. CISD provides a safe space for healthcare professionals to discuss their experiences and to support one another, and if implemented swiftly, may reduce the risk of developing long-term trauma-related disorders. Training staff on the frontline to act as debriefing facilitators can ensure that debriefing services are readily available to staff following a traumatic event.

Employee assistance programmes (EAPs) and psychological support services

Employee assistance programmes (EAPs) represent a crucial resource for providing confidential and accessible psychological support to healthcare professionals. Typically offering a range of services including confidential assessments, short-term counselling and referrals to mental health professionals where needed, EAPs can address a wide spectrum of work–life issues that contribute to stress and trauma, including family problems, financial or legal concerns and psychological challenges such as anxiety, depression and substance misuse.

Some EAPs also provide access to crisis intervention services and may facilitate CISDs following traumatic events in the workplace. Ensuring that healthcare professionals are well-informed about the availability of EAP services and how to access them is crucial. Organisations should also actively promote the confidential nature of these programmes to reduce any stigma associated with seeking psychological support.

Questions for reflection and discussion

1. What challenges do you recognise in implementing trauma-informed supervision in your work setting, and how might you work with colleagues, including those in leadership and management, to overcome these?
2. What level of recognition is there of STS and VT in your workplace? How can colleagues, supervisors and those in leadership and management be encouraged to look out for the effects of trauma on all staff, regardless of role or status?
3. How does your workplace encourage the self-awareness and self-care which are crucial for all clinicians, supervisors and managers? Identify why promoting these across the workforce is fundamental to implementing trauma-informed practice.
4. What difference might it make to patient outcomes where supervisors and managers, as well as individuals and the wider organisation, work in a trauma-informed way?
5. How can you promote compassionate and trauma-informed practice in your approach to yourself? How will it help you in your practice and in your supervision to be aware of your own triggers and of the ongoing impact of any past trauma?

Summary of learning points

This chapter has explored the following theoretical and practical approaches to supporting traumatised practitioners through self-awareness, supervision and reflective practice. Key points covered include:

- Self-awareness and the ability to engage in reflective practice as central to recognising our own emotional triggers and to enhancing our personal emotional regulation.

- Improved emotional regulation, as well as our ability to support colleagues, through taking care of our own needs.
- How STS and VT can lead to burnout, decreased job satisfaction and impaired clinical judgement.
- Trust, openness and freedom to be oneself as essential aspects of effective supervisory relationships, which are sometimes jeopardised in organisations that have a strong hierarchical structure and where TIC is not implemented.
- Where supervisors do not take a trauma-informed approach, this can lead to members of the workforce becoming increasingly traumatised through exposure to the traumas of those they work with – including patients, service users and colleagues.
- This underscores the need for trauma-informed supervision, which embeds safety, trustworthiness and transparency, collaboration, empowerment and choice.

Recommended follow-up reading

Bride, B.E., Sprang, G., Hendricks, A., Walsh, C.R., Mathieu, F., Hangartner, K., Ross, L.A., Fisher, P. and Miller, B.C. (2024). Principles for secondary traumatic stress-responsive practice: An expert consensus approach. *Psychological Trauma: Theory, Research, Practice, and Policy*, 16(8): 1301–1308.

Knight, C. and Borders, L.D. (2021). *Trauma-informed supervision: Core components and unique dynamics in varied practice contexts*. Abingdon: Routledge.

Getie, A., Ayenew, T., Amlak, B.T., Gedfew, M., Edmealem, A. and Kebede, W.M. (2025). Global prevalence and contributing factors of nurse burnout: An umbrella review of systematic review and meta-analysis. *BMC Nursing*, 24(1): 1–13.

Hansel, T.C. and Saltzman, L.Y. (2024). Secondary traumatic stress and burnout: The role of mental health, work experience, loneliness and other trauma in compassion fatigue in the healthcare workforces. *Traumatology*, 30(4): 615–618.

Najmabadi, L., Agénor, M. and Tendulkar, S. (2024). "Pouring from an empty cup": Manifestations, drivers, and protective factors of occupational stress among healthcare providers of trauma-informed care. *Journal of Interpersonal Violence*, 39(9/10): 2041–2075.

References

Al Barmawi, M., Shahrouri, B.E., Al Hadid, L., Alzoubi, M.M., Al-Mugheed, K., Alabdullah, A.A.S. and Abdelaliem, S.M.F. (2025). Measuring the prevalence, warning signs, and preventive measures of secondary traumatic stress among critical care nurses. *BMC Psychiatry*, 25: 450.

Berger, R. and Quiros, L. (2014). Supervision for trauma-informed practice. *Traumatology*, 20(4): 296–301.

Bouchard, L. and Rainbow, J. (2021). Compassion fatigue, presenteeism, adverse childhood experiences (ACES), and resiliency levels of doctor of nursing practice (DNP) students. *Nurse Education Today*, 100: 104852.

Burr, D., Alexander, L. and Searby, A. (2025). Perceived trauma among nurses during the COVID-19 pandemic: A qualitative descriptive study. *International Journal of Mental Health Nursing*, 34(2): 1–10.

Clark, C. and Aboueissa, A. (2021). Nursing students' adverse childhood experience scores: A national survey. *International Journal of Nursing Education Scholarship*, 18(1): 20210013.

Conti-O'Hare, M. (2002) *The nurse as wounded healer: From trauma to transcendence*. Burlington: Jones and Bartlett Learning.

Dar, I.A., Iqbal, N. and Emran, A. (2024). Secondary traumatic stress, vicarious posttraumatic growth, and rumination among healthcare professionals: Examining conditional indirect effect of secondary exposure to trauma. *Traumatology*, 30(3): 384–395.

Esaki, N. and Larkin, H. (2018). Prevalence of adverse childhood experiences (ACEs) among child service providers. *Families in Society*, 94(1): 31–37.

Esterhuizen, P. (2022). *Reflective practice in nursing* (Transforming nursing practice series). Thousand Oaks, CA: Learning Matters.

Harley, J. (2024). Developing self-awareness for effective nurse leadership. *Nursing Management - UK*, 31(5): 20–25.

Hazen, K.P., Carlson, M.W., Hatton-Bowers, H., Fessinger, M.B., Cole-Mossman, J., Bahm, J., Hauptman, K., Brank, E.M. and Gilkerson, L. (2020). Evaluating the facilitating attuned interactions (FAN) approach: Vicarious trauma, professional burnout, and reflective practice. *Children & Youth Services Review*, 112: 1–12.

HCPC. (2022). *Health and wellbeing framework*. https://www.hcpc-uk.org.uk/globalassets/resources/2022/health-and-wellbeing-framework-2022.pdf [Accessed 9th June 2025].

Jimenez, R.R., Andersen, S., Song, H. and Townsend, C. (2021). Vicarious trauma in mental health care providers. *Journal of Interprofessional Education & Practice*, 24: 1–5.

Kerasidou, A. (2019). Empathy and efficiency in healthcare at times of austerity. *Health Care Analysis*, 27(3): 171–184.

Markey, K., Murphy, L., O'Donnell, C., Turner, J. and Doody, O. (2020). Clinical supervision: A panacea for missed care. *Journal of Nursing Management*, 28(8): 2113–2117.

McGarva, K., Butler, H. and Newcombe, D. (2024). Insights towards trauma-informed nursing supervision: An integrative literature review and thematic analysis. *International Journal of Mental Health Nursing*.

Mercer, L., Cookson, A., Simpson-Adkins, G. and van Vuuren, J. (2023). Prevalence of adverse childhood experiences and associations with personal and professional factors in health and social care workers: A systematic review. *Psychological Trauma: Theory, Research, Practice and Policy*, 15(Suppl 2): S231–S245.

Morris, D.J., Webb, E.L., Kamath, S., Worsfold, J.J. and Dean, W. (2025). Looking beyond the frontline: Senior healthcare leaders' personal, professional and psychological experiences of the COVID-19 pandemic in the UK. *International Journal of Workplace Health Management*, 18(2): 219–237.

Mostafa, A.M.S., Wu, C.-H., Yunus, S., Deng, H. and Zaharie, M. (2025). Perceived abusive supervision and service performance: An attachment theory perspective. *Human Performance*, 38(2): 81–106.

Moudatsou, M., Stavropoulou, A., Philalithis, A. and Koukouli, S. (2020). The role of empathy in health and social care professionals. *Healthcare (Basel, Switzerland)*, 8(1): 26.

NMC. (2024). *Supporting information for reflection in nursing and midwifery practice*. nmc.org.uk/globalassets/sitedocuments/standards/supporting-information-for-reflection-in-nursing-and-midwifery-practice.pdf [Accessed 9th June 2025].

Nolte, A.G.W., Downing, C., Temane, A. and Hastings-Tolsma, M. (2017). Compassion fatigue in nurses: A metasynthesis. *Journal of Clinical Nursing*, 26: 4364–4378.

Noor, A.M., Suryana, D., Kamarudin, E.M.E., Naidu, N.B.M., Kamsani, S.R. and Govindasamy, P. (2025). Compassion fatigue in helping professions: A scoping literature review. *BMC Psychology*, 13(1): 1–22.

Prezerakos, P.E. (2018). Nurse managers' emotional intelligence and effective leadership: A review of the current evidence. *The Open Nursing Journal*, 12: 86–92.

Rabin, S., Kika, N., Lamb, D., Murphy, D.A.M., Stevelink, S., Williamson, V., Wessely, S. and Greenberg, N. (2023). Moral injuries in healthcare workers: What causes them and what to do about them? *Journal of Healthcare Leadership*, 15: 153–160.

RCN. (2024). *Self care*. rcn.org.uk/employment-and-pay/Health-safety-and-wellbeing/Self-care [Accessed 9th June 2025].

Rothwell, C., Kehoe, A., Farook, S.F. and Illing, J. (2021). Enablers and barriers to effective clinical supervision in the workplace: A rapid evidence review. *BMJ Open*, 11(9): e052929.

Safavi, H.P. and Bouzari, M. (2025). The deleterious effects of abusive supervision in health-care organizations. *Leadership in Health Services*. 1–16.

Sellers, T.P., LeBlanc, L.A. and Valentino, A.L. (2016). Recommendations for detecting and addressing barriers to successful supervision. *Behavior Analysis in Practice*, 9(4): 309–319.

Sist, L., Savadori, S., Grandi, A., Martoni, M., Baiocchi, E., Lombardo, C. and Colombo, L. (2022). Self-care for nurses and midwives: Findings from a scoping review. *Healthcare*, 10(12): 2473.

Sutton, L., Rowe, S., Hammerton, G. and Billings, J. (2022). The contribution of organisational factors to vicarious trauma in mental health professionals: A systematic review and narrative synthesis. *European Journal of Psychotraumatology*, 13(1): 2022278.

Vang, M.L. (2023). Indirect trauma exposure and secondary traumatization in health care: An individual or organizational problem? *Clinical Psychology: Science and Practice*, 30(3): 355–356.

Webb, E.L., Morris, D.J., Lupattelli Gencarelli, B. and Worsfold, J. (2024). The differential and accumulative impacts of self and other sources of moral injury on well-being in mental healthcare staff. *International Journal of Workplace Health Management*, 17(2): 139–155.

Williamson, V., Lamb, D., Hotopf, M., Raine, R., Stevelink, S., Wessely, S., Docherty, M., Madan, I., Murphy, D. and Greenberg, N. (2023). Moral injury and psychological wellbeing in UK healthcare staff. *Journal of Mental Health*, 32(5): 890–898.

Younas, A., Rasheed, S.P., Sundus, A. and Inayat, S. (2020). Nurses' perspectives of self-awareness in nursing practice: A descriptive qualitative study. *Nursing & Health Sciences*, 22(2): 398–405.

Conclusion

Sarah Housden

10

This concluding chapter aims to bring together the ideas and tools explored across the book by summarising the ground covered within a brief guide for best practice going forward.

1. Remain curious to the stories of patients and service users, listening to their narratives with open and empathic responses. Asking *'what is your story'* rather than *'what is wrong with you?'* is likely to establish a more trusting therapeutic relationship, which leads to constructive, healing and collaborative interactions, in which decision making can be shared and effective care plans can be co-constructed.

2. Recognise that traumas are more commonly experienced than we sometimes realise and that these may not always have been disclosed. In such situations, the impact and effects of trauma on the person's presentation may not have been identified within their clinical notes and medical records. Therefore, we need to avoid assuming that trauma has not been present in the person's distant or more recent past, just because there is no written record of it.

3. Be aware that traumas which occurred in childhood and adolescence have an impact across the lifespan. An individual's age does not exclude them from the ongoing effects of early-life traumas, and it is worth noting that suicide amongst older adults (over 65s) is correlated with adverse childhood events (Sachs-Ericsson et al., 2016). There is no age or time limit on the effect of trauma where effective restorative interventions have not been experienced.

4. Recognise that there is a link between mental and physical health. This is not always easily identified in a healthcare system that often separates

DOI: 10.4324/9781003635604-10

these two elements of experience and wellbeing. As healthcare practitioners, we will meet patients with physical symptoms without a known physical cause, sometimes identified as medically unexplained, somatic or psychosomatic symptoms. In these situations, it is possible that counselling or other psychotherapeutic approaches would be a better treatment option than physical interventions or medication. However, the certainty is that these symptoms are not likely to have been 'put on' or exaggerated by patients, and for the person living with fatigue and dizziness, chronic pain or sustained neurological symptoms in the absence of a physiological explanation, being or feeling disbelieved can add to their distress in marked and long-lasting ways.

5. As a healthcare worker, there is some likelihood that you and your colleagues will also have experienced trauma of some kind. It is important and helpful to pay attention to our own history and life experiences. By being aware of the part played by trauma in our own actions and interactions, we are more likely to be able to learn ways to recover, protect ourselves from ongoing exposure to traumatising events and experiences and to become increasingly resilient.

6. Consider the appropriateness of screening for trauma histories in some settings. This helps get a better understanding of the wider issues that might be bringing people to our services. However, avoid encouraging a detailed disclosure, which may be retraumatising, in a context where this cannot be quickly followed up on, or where the person cannot be supported in a sustained way. Remember that specialist services are there to offer psycho-therapeutic input, whereas the general nurse and allied health professional is more often able to act in signposting and information-providing ways, including supporting people to make small changes that can help them cope in the moment, until such time as specialist services can be accessed.

7. Listen to service users and patients, helping them find the words to express what might be happening for them. Be mindful of non-verbal communication and especially of appearing to be hurried as this is likely to be an invalidating experience and can take away from the value of anything your say.

8. Remain engaged with wider issues of equality and diversity, offering validation to service users and patients in a system that may have harmed them. This includes, for example, understanding the effects of racism and

widespread discrimination against those of low socio-economic, through disempowering systems and judgemental attitudes towards difference.

9. Remain mindful of the history patients and service users bring to the relationship and how past experiences might impact on the care we can provide. Be aware of the dangers of appearing to 'blame the victim' where an individual struggles to engage with services and service providers if they experience us as invalidating or triggering.

10. We can make a difference in our ability to develop meaningful relationships with our patients. Treisman (2016) notes that traumas which have occurred within broken relationships require healing within relationships. This is a message of hope for all clinicians. Every clinical encounter has the potential to be therapeutic; each communication is a chance to move closer to recovery and healing.

The tools in your toolkit

As this book draws to a close, it is worth reflecting upon the tools and techniques now available to you, along with knowledge and understanding of trauma, and ways to begin implementing trauma-informed care in your everyday healthcare practice and interactions with patients. Systems need to change too, with buy-in of organisational leaders and managers being essential to long-term, widespread and sustained implementation of trauma-informed approaches.

Amongst other approaches, you should now have a clear understanding of the need to listen to people's stories, supporting emotional grounding and slowing down breathing, as well as having ideas and suggestions for creating mental health 'rescue' toolkits. Together with encouraging ourselves and others to pay attention to the fundamentals of self-care to enhance all-round wellbeing, the importance of relationships and social aspects of health and wellbeing have been recognised, including regaining and maintaining work–life balance.

Furthermore, this book has aimed to provide you with an understanding of therapeutic approaches which whilst you are unlikely to implement with patients yourself, you may hear about or signpost them towards. These include dialectical behaviour therapy, trauma-focussed cognitive behavioural therapy and behavioural activation.

Finally, we can all be advocates for our patients as individuals, as well as at organisational and system levels. It is likely to be helpful going forward to spend time reflecting on what you have learned through reading this book, what actions you want to take forward for yourself from that learning and what you may want to share with and pass on to others, remembering that, truly, there is no 'them' and 'us' in healthcare.

References

Sachs-Ericsson, N.J., Rushing, N.C., Stanley, I.H. and Sheffler, J. (2016). In my end is my beginning: Developmental trajectories of adverse childhood experiences to late-life suicide. *Aging & Mental Health*, 20(2): 139–165.
Treisman, K. (2016). *Working with relational and developmental trauma in children and adolescents* (1st ed). London: Routledge.

Index

Note: Page numbers in *italics* and **bold** refer to figures and tables

abuse: child 33, 65; domestic 65; emotional 7, 11–12, 80, 83; parents 100; physical 7, 8, 12, 80, 111; sexual 8, 11, 12, 14, 29, 31, 80, 82, 92, 105, 110, 111; *see also* violence
achievement 87, 91–92
adolescence/adulthood 11, 14, 18, 31, 32, 36, 67–69, 93, 101, 155; *see also* child/childhood
adverse childhood experiences (ACEs) 1, 2, 7–8, 19, 20, 26–37, 101, 106, 107, 138; brain development and attachment 30–31; defined 28; healthcare practitioners 35–36; impact of 30–32, 35–36; lived experience of 33–34; overview 28; prevalence of 32–33; tools 34–35; *see also* trauma
advocate 19, 20, 33, 158
Agboola, I.K. 123
allied health professionals (AHPs) 7, 9, 16, 139; *see also* health/healthcare
anxiety 1, 8, 14, 31, 53–56, 92, 100, 103, 118, 119, 125, 136, 149; *see also* burnout; depression; mental health; stress; trauma
Asmussen, K. 33, 36
assessment 15, 52, 64, 119, 128, 130, 131, 136–137, 149

attachment 15; brain development and 30–31; defined 9–10; disorder 7; process of 10; theory 30–31; trauma 9–12; *see also* relationship
autonomic nervous system (ANS) 14
avoidance 47, 49, 57, 82, 87–89, 91–92, 128

Baca, K. 34
Bailey, Hannah 2
Baranowsky, A.B. 86
behaviour 49, 73, 80, 82, 83, 101; anti-social 14; brain and relational 15; coping 65, 69, 74; dismissive 106–107; health-harming 31, 36; PTSD 47
behavioural activation (BA) 87–90; benefits of 88; challenges of 89
Bellis, M. 30, 32
biosocial model 74
Black, Tamsin 2
Body, Achievement, Connection, Enjoyment and Spirituality (B.A.C.E.S) 78–95; achievement 91–92; BA 87–90; body care 91; connection 92–93; contemporary theory and practice 81–84; enjoyment 93; overview 80–81; reconnection 86; remembrance

and mourning 85–86; safety and stabilisation 85; self-soothing strategies 90; spirituality 93–94; tools 90; tri-phasic model 84–85
body care 91
borderline personality disorder (BPD) 68, 69, 83
boundaries 4, 72, 73, 141
Bowlby, J. 11, 30
brain 44–47, 46, 70, 71, 89, 104; development 11, 28, 29, 30–31, 66; and PTSD 44–47, 57; roles 44; see also adverse childhood experiences (ACEs)
breathing techniques 53–54, 54, 90; see also techniques
Bulford, E. 84, 129
burnout 126, 139, 145, 146, 149, 151; see also anxiety; compassion fatigue; depression; mental health; stress; trauma

care: choices 122; clinical 120; patients 108, 112, 143; self 68, 88, 89, 91, 93–95, 109, 145–147, 157
carers 34–36, 87, 122, 123, 125–126
Carvalho Silva, R. 12
case studies: abuse 4–6, 100–101; ACEs 26–27; C-PTSD 61–64; practitioner 136–137; PTSD 41–43; social services 78–80; TIC 118–119
Cherrill, Lou 2
child/childhood: abuse 33, 65; emotional abuse 11–12; violence/ obesity in 31; see also adolescence/ adulthood
children of alcoholics (COAs) 13
chronic stress 11, 14–16, 28, 29, 106, 111; see also stress
climate change 9
clinical practice 17, 32, 34, 69, 120
clinical supervision 138, 143
cognitive behavioural therapy for trauma (TF-CBT) 56, 57, 157

collaboration 81, 110, 121, 122, 125, 141, 142, 144, 151
colleagues feedback 147
communication 157; in healthcare supervision 143; non-verbal 72, 156; open 143–145, 149; skills 144, 145; workforce 142
compassion fatigue 139, 146; see also burnout
complex post-traumatic stress disorder (C-PTSD) 2, 11, 61–76, 81; adulthood 67–69; approaches 74–75; beginning of life 66–67; boundaries 72; listening skills 71; non-verbal communication 72; overview 64; patient in crisis 69–71; scenarios and events 65–66; therapy 73–74; tools 71–74; validation 72
connection 10, 12, 29, 30, 92–93, 108, 140, 148
contemporary theory and practice 81–84, 120–121, 138–140
Conti-O'Hare, M. 139
co-occurring conditions 51
coping behaviour 65, 69, 74; see also behaviour
coping strategies 16, 36, 56, 86, 88, 91, 109, 120, 122; see also mindfulness; professional development
COVID-19 pandemic 13, 103, 140
cow's milk protein allergy (CMPA) 41
critical incident stress debriefing (CISD) 149
critical incident stress management (CISM) 149

Delpierre, C. 8
Department of Health (DoH) 110
depression 8, 14, 15, 19, 31, 41, 49, 82, 83, 107, 123, 149; see also anxiety; burnout; stress; trauma
depressive symptoms 12, 68
developmental trauma 9–12; see also trauma

developmental trauma disorder (DTD) 7
Diagnostic and Statistical Manual of Mental Disorders, 5th Edition (DSM-5-TR) 7, 68
dialectical behaviour therapy (DBT) 73, 74
dismissive behaviour 106–107; *see also* behaviour
domestic violence 8, 29; *see also* violence

Elisseou, S. 126
emotional abuse 7, 11–12, 80; *see also* abuse
emotional distress 1–2, 87, 104
emotional dysregulation 7, 15–16, 69, 71, 75, 76
emotionally unstable personality disorder (EUPD) 7, 68, 83
emotional readiness 89
emotional regulation 34, 44, 66, 75, 104, 146, 150–151
empathy 12, 18, 126, 143, 145
employee assistance programmes (EAPs) 149–150
empowerment 81, 89, 110, 122–123, 141, 142, 144, 151
Emsley, E. 127
enjoyment 87, 93
Esaki, N. 139
Essential Mental Health Skills for Nurses and Allied Health Professionals 1, 3
eye movement desensitisation and reprocessing therapy (EMDR) 56, 57

Felitti, V. 29
Ford, K. 33, 34

gender 9, 13, 14, 53, 69, 123, 125, 132
Gentry, J.E. 86
Getting It Right for Every Child' (GIRFEC) 30
Gill, E. 32
Goldstein, E. 126

grounding techniques 54–55, 86, 90; *see also* techniques

health/health care 100–112; clinical supervision 143–144; impact on 31–32; physical 15, 28, 31, 36, 51, 105, 106, 108, 120, 125, 130, 155; practice 2, 109–110; practitioners 19, 34–36, 156; professionals 16–17; teams 33–34, 112, 125; worker 156; *see also* retraumatisation
Hedges, D.W. 44
Herman, J.L. 84–85
Hoeboer, C. 12
hyperarousal 14, 16, 50, 92
hypervigilance 15, 50, 57, 68, 81, 89, 92, 110, 111

International Classification of Diseases (ICD) 47, **48**, 50, 68
irritable bowel syndrome (IBS) 51
Isherwood, Trudii 2

Kaiser Permanente 28
Kelly-Irving, M. 8, 31
Kimberg, L.S. 90, 127
Kokokyi, S. 125
Kratzer, L. 16
Kulkarni, J. 69

Lamb, M.E. 83
language 6, 10, 12, 123
Larkin, H. 139
LGBTQIA+ 107
Linehan, M.M. 69, 74
listening skills 71; *see also* skills
lived experience 28, 33, 34
Lopez, M. 31, 33

Marmot, M. 9, 29, 32
Martin-Brown, Sharon 2
Maunder, R. 33
McLaughlin, K.A. 8

mental health 1–3, 15–16, 30, 92, 104–107, 111, 125, 139, 141, 149, 155, 157; *see also* anxiety; burnout
Mental Health Act 104, 111
Mercer, L. 33, 138
mindfulness 74, 147; *see also* coping strategies
Moran, Claire 2

National Association for People Abused in Childhood (NAPAC) 121, 122, 123
Nicki, A. 69
non-verbal communication 72, 156; *see also* communication
nurse/nursing 1, 2; and AHPs 16; clinical observations 70; triage 86; *see also* allied health professionals (AHPs); patients; trauma-informed care (TIC)

obesity 31
Olff, M. 9, 16

paradigm shift 108
parental violence 31; *see also* violence
Pargament, K.I. 94
patients 155, 156; care 108, 112, 143; in crisis 69–71; negative attitudes 143; stability 73–74; *see also* nurse/nursing; service user
personality disorder 12, 14, 63, 64, 65, 67–70, 74, 75, 83, 107
physical abuse 7, 8, 12, 80, 111; *see also* abuse
physical health 15, 28, 31, 36, 51, 105, 106, 108, 120, 125, 130, 155; *see also* health/healthcare
physiological responses 14–15
Positive and Proactive Care: reducing the need for restrictive interventions 110
post-traumatic growth 87
post-traumatic stress disorder (PTSD) 2, 7, 11, 41–58, 111, 139; avoidance 49; brain and 44–47, *46*; breathing

techniques 53–54; co-occurring conditions 51; grounding techniques 54–55; interventions for 55–56; overview 43; perception of threat 50; re-experiencing 48–49; reframing thoughts 55; self-management skills 53; symptoms/wellbeing 47–51; tools 51–55
poverty 9, 13, 20, 29, 32, 105
practitioner: CISM 149; clinical supervision 143–144; contemporary theory and practice 138–140; EAPs 149–150; healthy work–life balance 146; ideas for longer-term 148–150; managing emotional reactions 146–147; managing stress and trauma 147; overview 137–138; personal resilience 147–148; reflective practice 141; reflective supervision 141–143; self-awareness 140–141; support colleagues with trauma 144–146; tools 146–148; traumatised 136–151
professional development 3, 143, 148; *see also* coping strategies
psychiatric disorders 12, 15, 83
psychological trauma 6–8, 34, 111, 139; *see also* trauma; trauma-informed care (TIC)
psychotraumatology 9

racial trauma 13; *see also* trauma
racism 8, 13, 20, 156–157
Read, A. 87
reconnection 86
reduce stigma 69, 108, 123
re-experiencing 44, 47–49
reflection 3, 18, 141, 143, 145
reflective practice 141–142, 150
reflective supervision 138, 141–142, 148, 149
relational trauma 9–12; *see also* trauma
relationship: building trust in 11, 19, 20; positive 35, 36; supervisory 138,

142–144, 151; therapeutic 72, 85, 102, 107–108, 111, 121, 126, 155; *see also* attachment
remembrance and mourning 85–86
resilience 9, 16, 19, 81, 148; emotional 141; enhancing personal 147–148; personal 147–148
restrictive interventions 104, 110–112
retraumatisation 100–112; dismissive attitudes 106–107; features of 102–106; healthcare practice 109–110; overview 101–102; recovery steps 108; restrictive interventions 110–112; self care 109; therapeutic relationship 107–108; tools 108–110
Rothwell, C. 142
Ryan, R. 31

safety 121; physical and psychological 109, 149; and stabilisation 85; trust and 34, 85
Salsbury, S. 34
Scottish Health Network 30
secondary traumatic stress (STS) 138, 151
self-awareness 138, 140–141
self-care 68, 88, 89, 91, 93–95, 109, 145–147, 157; *see also* care
self-management skills 53; *see also* skills
self-reflection 139, 147
self-regulation techniques 147; *see also* techniques
self-soothing 55, 85, 90
service user 1–3, 13, 17–18, 56, 69, 71, 81, 82, 90, 110, 122, 123, 125, 130, 137–138, 155–157; *see also* patients
sexual abuse 8, 11, 12, 14, 29, 31, 80, 82, 92, 105, 110, 111; *see also* abuse
sexual violence 7, 85; *see also* violence
Simons, M. 125
skills 74; based approach 73; communication 144, 145; listening 71; for practice 3; reframing thoughts

55; self-management 53; self-nurturing 145; telephone coaching 74
social anxiety 92, 100; *see also* anxiety
social connections 93, 147
social interaction 49, 66, 92, 103, 104
Sodal, E. 34
SOLER 72
spirituality 87, 93–94
staff members 121, 126, 127, 145
stress 10, 14, 15, 47, 106, 111, 146–149; *see also* anxiety; burnout; depression; mental health
structural stigma, defined 107
structural trauma 13–14; *see also* trauma
Substance Abuse and Mental Health Services Administration (SAMHSA) 120, 121, 127, 130
Sweeney, A. 84, 127
systemic trauma 13–14; *see also* trauma

techniques: breathing 53–54, *54*; for enhancing resilience 148; grounding 54–55, 86, 90; self-regulation 147; self-soothing 55, 85, 90; tools and 56
therapeutic relationship 72, 85, 102, 107–108, 111, 121, 126, 155; *see also* relationship
threat, perception of 50
trauma 4–21, 94; attachment/relational/ developmental 9–12; defined 7; effects of 14–16; emotional dysregulation and mental health 15–16; experiences 9–14; health professionals 16–17; of neglect 12–13; overview 6; physiological responses 14–15; reducing and managing 18–20; secondary 2, 139; systemic/structural 13–14; tools 17–18; *see also* anxiety; burnout; depression; psychological trauma
trauma-informed care (TIC) 1, 2, 82, 85, 118–131, **124**; approach 120, 130–131; barriers 127–129; benefits of 123–127; carers 125–126;

choices 122; collaboration 122;
contemporary theory and practice
120–121; cultural/historical/gender
considerations 123; empowerment
122–123; enquiring 129–130;
healthcare practice 109–110;
implementation of 127; organisation
128; overview 119–120; principles
of 121–123, 142; safety 121; service
users 125; staff members 126; tools
129–130; trustworthiness 121–122;
see also psychological trauma
Treisman, K. 157
tri-phasic model 84–85
trustworthiness 121–122, 141, 142,
144, 151
Turner, Rebecca 2

Valeras, A.B. 34
validation 18, 53, 72, 93, 110, 156
vicarious trauma (VT) 138, 151; *see
also* trauma

victim 8, 11, 16, 29, 80, 82, 106; blame
148, 157; PTSD 82; sexual abuse
110; of sexual assault 103, 109
violence: domestic 8; family or
community 7; parental 31; sexual 7,
85; *see also* abuse
Violence Against Women and Girls
(VAWG) 13
vulnerability 10, 16, 81, 88, 91, 93
Vygotsky, L.S. 10

Waite, R. 31
Walker, P. 69
wellbeing 2, 12, 31, 47–51, 81, 88,
103, 105, 141, 145–148, 157
Winnicott, D.W. 66–67
Woon, F.L. 44
workforce 28, 35, 85, 131, 139, 142,
144, 146
World Health Organization (WHO) 7, 9

Zanarini, M.C. 83

For Product Safety Concerns and Information please contact our EU
representative GPSR@taylorandfrancis.com
Taylor & Francis Verlag GmbH, Kaufingerstraße 24, 80331 München, Germany

www.ingramcontent.com/pod-product-compliance
Lightning Source LLC
Chambersburg PA
CBHW050608280326
41932CB00016B/2962